"*Sex, Social Justice, and Intimacy in Mental Health Practice* identifies the lack of sexual health education in graduate school training programs as a social justice issue. The author challenges the mental health field to create greater access to sexual health services, services that have historically been reserved only for the privileged. Sharing information, cases, and activities from her years of work as both a clinician/sex therapist and an educator, Martinez-Gilliard offers a comprehensive guide to sexual health competency that is a must for any training program wanting to prepare its students to meet the holistic needs of clients and to create a healthier society."

Prem Pahwa, LMSW, CST; *Director of The University of Michigan Sexual Health Certificate Program*

"Bridging previous work across sexuality, psychology, social work, and other allied fields, Erin Martinez-Gilliard offers an intentional and compassionate guide to everything from building rapport that allows for talk about sexuality to diagnosing sexual challenges, plus a bevy of potential tools and intervention options alongside case studies to support a deeper understanding of how to utilize them."

Shanna K. Kattari, PhD, MEd, CSE, ACS; *Associate Professor, University of Michigan; Pronouns: They/Them/Theirs*

Sex, Social Justice, and Intimacy in Mental Health Practice

This book aims to equip mental health professionals to integrate discussions of sexual identity, health, wellness, and intimacy into the scope of their client's mental health, ensuring they are well-prepared to incorporate sexual functioning into core assessment, interventions, and treatment.

We exist in societies that are scared to discuss sexual health, identity, and relationships, and the stigma surrounding these topics saturates our mental health professions. Sex, intimacy, and sexual identity have historically been relegated as "specialized" topics when training new clinicians, which has led to professionals feeling unable and unskilled to speak about a core part of their client's psychological, biological, physical, and relational health. Viewing this as a social justice issue, this book addresses a movement in the counseling field to incorporate sexual health into therapy as well as providing new ways of foundational teaching. Chapters begin exploring the history of sex therapy and the problems that have previously been addressed as concerns for the sex therapy field only, before discussing issues surrounding transference and countertransference. Encouraging self-reflection regarding values, bias, and attitudes related to topics of sexuality, the book moves to discussing strategies and integrative approaches to co-occurring conditions, such as trauma, diagnosis of sexual difficulties, stigma and societal messages, biopsychosocial treatment, networking, and coordination of care and spiritual health and healing.

Including journaling exercises, assessment tools and case studies of how to weave approaches addressing sexual concerns into practice, this book will provide graduate courses and continuing education instructors with the core material to assist the training and development of future and established professionals.

Erin Martinez-Gilliard is a certified sex therapist, clinical social worker and lecturer at the University of Michigan, School of Social Work. She is dedicated to increasing access to sex therapy and trauma-informed treatment in mental health services.

Sex, Social Justice, and Intimacy in Mental Health Practice

Incorporating Sexual Health in Approaches to Wellness

ERIN MARTINEZ-GILLIARD

Routledge
Taylor & Francis Group

NEW YORK AND LONDON

Designed cover image: © Getty Images

First published 2023
by Routledge
605 Third Avenue, New York, NY 10158

and by Routledge
4 Park Square, Milton Park, Abingdon, Oxon, OX14 4RN

Routledge is an imprint of the Taylor & Francis Group, an informa business

ISBN: 978-0-367-76133-2 (hbk)
ISBN: 978-0-367-76312-1 (pbk)
ISBN: 978-1-003-16638-2 (ebk)

DOI: 10.4324/9781003166382

Typeset in Dante and Avenir
by Apex CoVantage, LLC

This book is dedicated to my mom and dad for helping me value and pursue learning, my husband for supporting my writing, and my son for constantly inspiring me.

Contents

Introduction

While writing this book the United States has seen sexual health and human rights attacked on a horrifying level with the United States Supreme Court overturning Roe vs. Wade in July 2022, multiple states barring gender affirming care for children and adolescents and the banning of books and education that acknowledge the existence of sexual orientation and gender diversity. The basic right to be seen, to exist, is being taken away in several states within the country. Basic medical care, the choice of how to best care for one's body, is no longer available to millions of individuals. Parents, social workers, medical professionals and teachers are also at increased risk in this terrifying era we have entered. Offering education or services about identity, bodies, and sexual health is no longer legal in several states and could result in loss of professional licenses, harassment, prosecution, and imprisonment.

Sharing the information in this book has always felt important to me. Sexual rights are human rights. Sexual justice is social justice. Incorporating sexual health in our mental health services is not a specialty; rather, it is a foundational part of the work. Throughout my career I have witnessed many people's discomfort with the topic, resulting in dismissive comments, minimizing the importance of the topic, refusing to offer training or courses on the topic or shaming those who do discuss it. It has often been a fight to ensure individuals have access to information about their sexual selves. This fight is even more present, more crucial, and more consequential than ever before. This fight belongs to all of us.

I began my social work career long before graduate school. I didn't know anything about the field of social work and I had a strong dislike for therapy

DOI: 10.4324/9781003166382-1

settings. As a teenager, therapists had created my narrative versus listening to me and empowering my story. I felt unsafe and unheard in those spaces. At 19 years old, I was a case manager with a caseload of nearly 150 women. I usually worked 10–12-hour days buried in systems beside the families that lived in the rubble of these systems. I ended every day with feelings of exhaustion, inspiration, curiosity, pain, and hope.

I met Betty, a 40-something single mom and grandma. She had survived a major open-heart surgery a few years back, leaving a long scar on her chest. She worked hard each day to stay free of heroin after more than a decade of IV use. Her laughter and stories were too great a distraction from my endless paperwork. Despite my naïve presentation and lack of life experience, Betty welcomed me into her story. Working caregiving jobs at the time, Betty dreamed of being an exotic dancer. Despite scars from track lines on her arms, several missing teeth and an enormous scar from open-heart surgery, Betty knew she was sexy. I worried about her ability to be able to be successful and safe in this type of setting. I wondered why Betty believed she would enjoy this type of work. She told me she loved the idea of the stage and being seen. She saw the dance and the stage as a place she would hold control and direct their gaze as she wanted. Betty embodied resilience. She had experienced so many traumatic events over the course of her life. To believe she could dance, to believe she was sexy, was to have hope and demand the right to pleasure. It was also her way of rewriting the narrative of the beauty of her body and relationship to her body.

I met Angel, a 22-year-old mother to baby girl twins. I kept a blanket in my office for Angel. She often fell asleep with her head on the desk as we attempted to complete paperwork. She was very sick with AIDS. As a runaway she had survived through sex work, likely contracting HIV in her early teen years. She said she was bitter that sex would kill her when it had never brought her pleasure, despite hundreds of sexual experiences in her short lifetime.

And later in my career. . . .

I met Cortez in juvenile residential placement for committing a sexual assault. At only 15 years old he was away from family and community in a medium-secure facility after sexually abusing two younger cousins. During his time in placement, he shared memories of being five or six years old and watching his mother be raped and abused. He also discussed several boyfriends of his mother who physically and sexually abused him. In placement he struggled to find regulation in his behavior. Compulsive masturbation was a common treatment issue. He wondered if he could ever be healthy and have a girlfriend and "behave like normal."

It seems that the hundreds of people that filled my early professional life pointed me in the direction of sex therapy. I currently work as a clinical social worker and

AASECT-certified sex therapist in an out-patient mental health practice. I am also a teaching professor at the University of Michigan School of Social Work. I am in a place in my career where I have so many wonderful tools to help assess and understand how sexual pleasure, pain, trauma, and intimacy are woven into the presenting problems and biopsychosocial understanding of my clients. I have many interventions and safe ways to have meaningful conversations around sexual health and a wonderful network of providers to support the work. I also am well aware that my initial education and training did not prepare me to ask the right questions, create a healing and safe space for myself or my clients, and certainly didn't offer interventions that touched sexuality, identity, and intimacy.

I am deeply sorry for the ways my lack of interventions failed Betty, Angel, and Cortez. I am so grateful for their honesty and insight in sharing their stories. They refused to allow me to see them as anything less than their full identities, including their sexual selves. I offer many of the concepts and tools I have learned along the way in this book for developing mental health professionals. I hope this book is a safe and approachable way to expand your comfort and knowledge in the content of sexuality and intimacy in social work and other mental health professions. We deserve ways to be comfortable and informed in this topic. The vast majority of graduate, educational settings are extremely limited in addressing sex, sexuality, and intimacy as a foundational topic of wellness and mental health. In this, they contribute to the secrecy and stigma, that keeps individuals from freely knowing themselves, continues violence and disease and sometimes death. Sexuality and social work are not an elective but foundational to coursework.

Betty and Angel are no longer with us. I am grateful for the way Betty, Angel, and many other beautiful people bravely and patiently taught me how to fully be in this work. I hope this book brings discomfort that is essential to growth and confidence in tools that open conversations and self-knowledge for your clients and future clients.

In each chapter of this book, you will find case examples to demonstrate the concepts and tools in a realistic manner.

The following is one more beautiful human being that shared her story with me early in my career. We will check in with Roseanna at the end of the book.

Case Example – Roseanna

Roseanna is a cisgender, Latinx woman in her early 30s. She identifies as bisexual. She describes being self-employed as a sex worker for approximately a decade. I meet Roseanna as a clinical social worker at a domestic violence and sexual assault program that offers short-term, free-of-cost counseling services. During the first few minutes of meeting, she sees me glance at her intake paperwork that she completed over the phone with the crisis team. She shrugs and shares that the information won't be that helpful because she had to make a few things up in order to get the appointment. I am curious and ask for her to elaborate. Roseanna shares that if she presents as having fears and concerns about being a sex worker, most programs are more likely to see her deserving of services, but she actually wants help related to sexual pleasure.

One part of the intake paperwork that she states is accurate is the history of mental health services. She has attempted to address this presenting problem with four different mental health professionals in the last three years. She shares that her problem was consistently viewed as an invalid concern and that her employment as a sex worker was considered a trauma history worthy of focus in therapy. Roseanna is clear with me that she is happy to discuss her experience as a sex worker but would prefer to focus on the presenting problem of lack of orgasm (DSM Diagnosis: F52.3 Orgasmic Disorder) throughout her lifetime.

Roseanna's difficulty in receiving treatment sounds very familiar. I respect the creativity she has used to navigate a flawed mental health system in order to receive treatment. She describes the symptoms of anorgasmia as causing difficulties in her intimate, romantic relationships. She shares that she has always felt like something is missing from her life because she has been unable to experience an orgasm. She feels a sense of sadness and hopelessness in this part of her life. She also feels a sense of disconnect from her own body as a result of this problem. Her ideal treatment would allow her to explore this issue from a biological and psychological approach. She would like to gain insight into her relationship with her body as well as partnered, intimate experiences. She would like to learn approaches to sexual experiences that may increase the potential for orgasm.

Roseanna is insightful and her hopes for treatment are well-aligned with basic components of sex therapy. If she shared that divorce, job loss, a traumatic event, was causing her relational difficulties, with symptoms of sadness and hopelessness, I would be well-trained to offer an informed treatment plan. Her presenting concern would never be seen as invalid or unworthy of treatment. Despite sexual health, intimacy, and connection to one's own body being core to wellness, medical, and mental health professionals often receive little to no training to address this in treatment. Programs to address these core components of a person's life are considered "specialized." The services that Roseanna needs then become very much out of her reach. They often exist in affluent communities and many services are private-pay only or are covered by limited commercial insurances. For Roseanna, who works extremely hard for a living wage and receives Medicaid, specialized services are not available or affordable.

What this book will provide and what it does not intend to provide:

As a teacher, I am reminded of the intense feeling of responsibility held by students embarking on their social work career. The fear of not knowing "enough" (often expressed as the desire to be educated in everything), often results in demands and desires to have all of the information about all the diagnosis' problems and concerns that may meet us at the doors of our clinical spaces. As graduation approaches, anxiety often ramps up and I must deliver the hard news:

You will not know all you need to know to help your future clients when you leave this program. You should be well-prepared to connect and conduct a thorough biopsychosocial assessment to diagnosis disorders based on an understanding of presenting problems and symptoms. You should understand many clinical modalities and be able to apply the modalities to build intervention plans.

Just as I share this with students leaving the safety of the classroom and entering into the enormous responsibility of clinical work, I share this with you, the reader.

This book hopes to provide you with (1) the ethical framework to inspire you to always incorporate sexual health and intimacy work into your standard assessment and treatment approach, (2) the comfort and skill to open the conversation with all clients and (3) tools to apply to many presenting problems that will increase insight and confidence. This book will also make you more aware of what you do not know related to sexuality and sexual health work.

There are several amazing books about sexual health in the mental health profession. I recommend many as reference books for mental health professionals. This book will not offer the same type of detailed overview on an extensive list of topics related to sexual health. I have written this book in the same method that I teach, diving deep into case examples to illustrate assessment and intervention tools. Each chapter offers language to introduce and explore topics as well as several step-by-step instructions for specific tools. This book will also help you reflect on some of your own values, bias, and fears that surround the topic of sexuality.

I hope this book does not simply expose you to concepts and information but rather provides you with the language, inspiration, and tools to use this material with clients. You will not be an expert or define yourself as a sex therapist after reading this book, but you will be very capable of exploring and understanding a client's sexuality and concerns related to sexual intimacy. You will be able to provide resources to address concerns, as well as have an understanding of why the difficulties exist and the short-term goals needed to improve them. One of the first trainings I attended on the topic of sex therapy was titled "Why Talking About Sex Will Change The World." I hope this book will allow you to begin this important work of changing the world. There is a lot of work to do!

The Social Injustice of Specialization

1

Introduction

Sex therapy is a modality within the field of psychotherapy. It includes topics of sexual health and more deeply incorporates sexuality as an emotional and relational aspect of the person. Sexuality and issues of intimacy are core to the human experience across the lifespan. It is an integral part of wellness. Strangely, it is often overlooked or avoided in client sessions and graduate-level courses.

Overview of Sex Therapy Field

The sex therapy field dates back centuries. Research in the field has historically been difficult because most cultures viewed sex as a private issue that was inappropriate to discuss. Researchers who attempted to discuss it, even when related to a medical, psychological or sociological lens, were often determined perverse.

In Western cultures we are most familiar with the research of Henry Havelock Ellis, whose work in co-authoring the first medical textbook on "homosexuality," as well as published works on sex practices, influenced the field in the early 1900s. Alfred Kinsey, biologist, zoologist, and sexologist of Indiana University, had a strong influence on the field of sexual health. He and his team of researchers interviewed approximately 18,000 individuals on their sex histories, resulting in the publications known as The Kinsey Reports.

DOI: 10.4324/9781003166382-2

Kinsey is also known for the Kinsey Scale, a rating scale of heterosexuality and homosexuality that encouraged the view of orientation expression as a continuum versus a binary. Kinsey's teaching and research took place in the early to mid-1900s (Drucker, 2010).

While earlier research sought to understand both common and "deviant" sex behaviors, the field transitioned to defining sexual problems and understanding them more thoroughly in the mid-19th century. William Masters and Virginia Johnson, commonly Masters and Johnson, are credited for their work in studying individual and couples' sexual response. Their direct observation of more than 600 individuals engaged in sexual experiences resulted in detailed information about the anatomical and physiological process. This information resulted in what is defined as the Human Sexual Response: Excitement, Plateau, Orgasm, Resolution. The move from interviews to laboratory study substantiated the field of sexology and also moved the field to a more medicalized view of sexuality (Levin, 2008).

The idea of sexual dysfunction, defined by symptoms and the inability to "respond" sexually, according to the response cycle, was originally researched and defined by Masters and Johnson and remains the standard assessment of the field. Medical professionals and mental health professionals evaluating presenting problems of sexual experiences rely on the Diagnostic and Statistical Manual of Disorders (DSM-5-TR) and The International Classification of Diseases (ICD 11). Within the DSM-5-TR sexual dysfunctions include:

Delayed Ejaculation

The inability to achieve ejaculation despite the presence of adequate sexual stimulation and the desire to ejaculate.

Erectile Disorder

The repeated failure to obtain or maintain erections during partnered sexual activities.

Female Orgasmic Disorder

The difficulty experiencing orgasm and/or markedly reduced intensity of orgasmic sensations.

Female Interest/Arousal Disorder

An absence or reduced frequency or intensity in interest in sexual activity, absent/reduced erotic thoughts, no/reduced initiation of sexual activity, absent/reduced sexual excitement during sexual activity, absent/reduced sexual interest/arousal in response to internal or external sexual/erotic cues, absent/reduced genital or non-genital sensations during sexual activities (three or six of symptoms must be present)

Genito-Pelvic Pain/Penetration Disorder

A persistent difficulty with vaginal penetration, vulvovaginal/pelvic pain during intercourse or penetration attempts, anxiety about pain in anticipation or during vaginal penetration or tightening of pelvic floor muscles during attempted vaginal penetration. (1 of these symptoms must be present)

Male Hypoactive Disorder

A low/absent desire for sex and deficient/absent sexual thoughts fantasies

Premature (Early) Ejaculation

A persistent or recurrent pattern of ejaculation during partnered sexual activity within approximately 1 minute following vaginal penetration and before individual wishes it (diagnosis may involve penetration other than vagina but criteria not established for other types of penetration).

Substance/Medication-Induced Sexual Dysfunction

A clinically significant disturbance in sexual function developed during or soon after substance intoxication or withdrawal or after exposure to a medication (American Psychiatric Association, 2022).

These definitions are rarely how clients present problems; rather, the disorders are based on biological difficulties with psychological, emotional, and relational underpinnings.

Specific sexual symptoms occur within phases of the Human Sexual Response Cycle. The Human Sexual Response Cycle was originally defined by Masters and Johnson and revised by sex therapist Helen Singer Kaplan in 1979. Kaplan added the phase desire, highlighting that one of the most common sexual problems is the lack of desire. The following diagram, Figure 1.1, illustrates the relationship of symptoms (sexual dysfunction) with specific diagnosis. These symptoms occur within specific phases of the response cycle (Levin, 2008).

In a mental health setting, I use the human sexual response cycle and diagnostic criteria to determine where in the experience of sexual activity an individual is having difficulty. If we consider:

Roseanna (from our introduction) shares that she experiences sexual interest *(desire phase)* in the form of fantasy for her partner. After sexual engagement is initiated, she notes that her body responds in ways known in the Human Sexual Response Cycle as *excitement*. However, her frustration is that despite "feeling close to it," she has never orgasmed. Depending on my clinical setting, I may complete the assessment for Female Orgasmic Disorder, but what seems most important is that I have used her description of the problem along with the data and criteria to narrow down the problem. More to come on how we can address this with Roseanna.

It is important that we understand how differently these difficulties are presented outside a diagnostic text. We will learn more about that in future chapters as well as how to enter conversations and ask questions that help us to better understand the presenting problem.

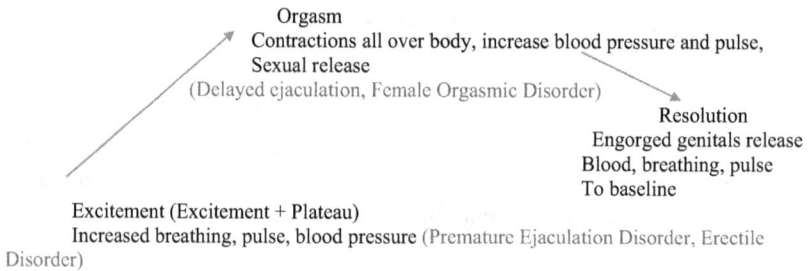

Orgasm
Contractions all over body, increase blood pressure and pulse, Sexual release
(Delayed ejaculation, Female Orgasmic Disorder)

Resolution
Engorged genitals release
Blood, breathing, pulse
To baseline

Excitement (Excitement + Plateau)
Increased breathing, pulse, blood pressure (Premature Ejaculation Disorder, Erectile Disorder)

Desire:
Genitals engorge with blood, penis enlarges, vagina expands, sexual flush, nipple erection, uterus ascends, scrotal tightening and lifting (Erectile Disorder, Female sexual interest/arousal disorder, Male hypoactive sexual desire disorder)
** Substance/medication-induced sexual dysfunction and Genito Pelvic Pain/Penetration Disorder could present in any of the phases of response.

Figure 1.1 Sexual Response Cycle and Associated Diagnosis

Social Justice and Sexual Health

Sexual health is a topic that is often feared, shamed, privatized, and, more recently, specialized. In order for an individual to experience sexual health, our organizations and services must consider sexual health as an entity that spans the biological, psychological, spiritual, and emotional realms of an individual's life.

The Sexuality Information and Education Council of the United States (SIECUS) has developed the Guidelines for Comprehensive Sexuality Education for over a decade. These Guidelines were developed by a variety of experts from the U.S. Centers for Disease Control and Prevention, the American Medical Association, the National School Boards Association, the National Education Association, the March of Dimes Birth Defects Foundation and Planned Parenthood Federation of America, as well as school-based sexuality education teachers, national program developers and experienced trainers. The Guidelines offer support to schools and communities to develop and evaluate their sexual health curriculums for children/youth, from kindergarten through twelfth grade.

SEICUS Guidelines are built around six key concepts surrounding sexuality. The guidelines encompass much more than abstinence or condoms; they expand learning and understanding to culture, values, consent, and relationships. These six key concept areas are:

> **Key Concept 1**: Human Development. Human development is characterized by the interrelationship between physical, emotional, social, and intellectual growth.
>
> **Key Concept 2**: Relationships. Relationships play a central role throughout our lives.
>
> **Key Concept 3**: Personal Skills. Healthy sexuality requires the development and use of specific personal and interpersonal skills.
>
> **Key Concept 4**: Sexual Behavior. Sexuality is a central part of being human and individuals express their sexuality in a variety of ways.
>
> **Key Concept 5**: Sexual Health. The promotion of sexual health requires specific information and attitudes to avoid unwanted consequences of sexual behavior.
>
> **Key Concept 6**: Society and Culture. Social and cultural environments shape the way individuals learn about and express their sexuality.
>
> (Sexuality Information and Education Council of the
> United States, 2004)

These guidelines illustrate the importance of comprehensive sexuality education and exploration. When we work with clients, we can assume that the vast majority of individuals have not experienced this type of education and exploration about themselves in family, in community or in schools. Sex education curricula in the United States that are considered "progressive" are often those that offer information about contraception versus abstinence-only education. Very rarely do we consider individual's right to pleasure as key to education.

The term "intimate justice," developed by Psychologist Sarah McClelland, requires that we understand the role of expectation related to sexual fulfillment. McClelland states that beliefs about one's self and one's future sexual self are influenced by three specific dimensions: the socio-political conditions of sexual development, psychological self-evaluation processes and norms concerning the distribution of justice (McClelland, 2010).

In research and in medical and clinical spaces we grossly minimize and simplify satisfaction or pleasure into broad statements such as, "are you sexually satisfied?" Access to information about ourselves, the representation of ourselves as sexual beings in media, education, policy, and medicine, influences our view of ourselves and what we imagine as possible for our sexual lives. Social stigma and access to information limits intimate justice for many groups. As clinicians we have the opportunity to either open the dialogue or continue in silence and limitation.

Using the Sexual Health Assessment in Chapter 5, we will learn ways to introduce a more encompassing view of sexuality for each client that allows them access to intimate justice. This work is necessary rather than a specialized service or "add on" as it is often treated in many agencies and private practices. The ethical code of Social Work upholds two major principles and values directly addressing incorporating the full human being into the consideration of services to develop intervention as well as ensuring access to information and basic health.

These values and ethical principles are defined as:

Value: Social Justice

Ethical Principle: Social workers challenge social injustice

The National Association of Social Workers (NASW) defines this ethical principle as the need to "pursue social change, particularly with on behalf of vulnerable and oppressed individuals and groups of people. . . . Social workers strive to ensure access to needed information, services, and resources;

equality of opportunity; and meaningful participation in decision making for all people."

Value: Dignity and Worth of the Person

Ethical Principle: Social workers respect the inherent dignity and worth of the person.

NASW defines this ethical principle as the need to "treat each person in a caring and respectful fashion, mindful of individual differences and cultural and ethnic diversity. Social workers promote clients socially responsible self-determination. Social workers seek to enhance clients' capacity and opportunity to change and to address their own needs" (Workers, 2008).

The World Health Organization (WHO) also offers a broad definition of sexuality and sexual rights as components of socially-just services throughout the world. Defining sex, sexual health, sexuality, and sexual rights began in 1974 and resulted in these working definitions through coordinated work with the Pan American Health Organization (2000):

> Sexual health cannot be defined, understood or made operational without a broad consideration of sexuality, which underlies important behaviors and outcomes related to sexual health. The working definition of sexuality is:
>
> > "a central aspect of being human throughout life encompasses sex, gender identities and roles, sexual orientation, eroticism, pleasure, intimacy, and reproduction. . . . Sexuality is influenced by the interaction of biological, psychological, social, economic, political, cultural, legal, historical, religious, and spiritual factors."
> >
> > (Weston, 2004)

As trained mental health practitioners we learn to assess health and well-being from a psychological, biological, relational, and spiritual perspective. Through a collaborative relationship with our clients, we create a consensual, safe space to learn about current functioning and history within these domains. While the biopsychosocial assessment is foundational to most education and supervision for mental health professionals, the inclusion of sexuality and intimacy is inconsistent in the assessment. When terms such as sexual history, sexuality, and sexual relationships are included in assessment and intervention documents, it is often addressed in a limited and sometimes negative fashion. In 25 years of practice, I have reviewed hundreds of initial assessment documents and countless times I have seen this domain completed with comments such as, "client does not report any sexual partners," or "there is no history of sexual abuse," or "client is married and does not have concerns about sex at this time." It seems that mental health practitioners often do not understand what should be discussed surrounding the topics of sexuality and intimacy.

A sexual health assessment, used as a standard document of assessment in sex therapy, seeks to gain information about:

> How an individual views themselves and feels about themselves as a sexual person
>
> The history of values/beliefs related to sexual identity
>
> Formative experiences related to sexual identity
>
> How an individual cares for their sexual needs and sexual health
>
> How an individual currently experiences sexual pleasure,
>
> How an individual hopes to experience sexual pleasure in the future and how they have experienced it in the past (what has changed and why)
>
> What education have they received about their body and sexual care for their body
>
> What myths or misinformation influences their belief regarding caring for their body
>
> Have they had and do they currently have access to tools for safe and pleasurable sexual experiences (lubrication, contraception, condoms, dental dams, devices for sexual play).

Key to this collaborative process of exploring sexuality and intimacy is understanding how a person knows what they know, as well as their history which influences values, beliefs, and behaviors. Understanding what a person knows also helps the mental health practitioner to consider the space between current functioning and their goals, as well as what is needed to bridge that gap. For some clients, this may be about education or resources, and for others this may be related to exploration of identity, family history or sexual experiences. The domain of sexuality and intimacy is integrated with biological, psychological, relational, and spiritual health and well-being. When we understand functioning in this domain, we are able to develop a holistic view of the client and treatment goals that are more accurate to the individual's lived experience. Let's take a look a simple case example.

Lizette seeks mental health services related to a consistent sad mood that she has been experiencing for approximately three months. She notes low motivation and decreased energy. There is a sense of fatigue and decreased engagement in formerly pleasurable activities.

Biological: Lizette does not report any health concerns. She has a daily routine that includes access to healthy foods and exercise opportunities. She uses substances in a limited fashion (one to two times a month) and does not rely on marijuana or alcohol to modify mood. She would like to lose a few pounds to fit into some of the clothes she wore in a past season and feels if her motivation and energy increases, this will be possible. Psychological: Lizette reports feeling less motivation and energy in the last several months. She often feels sad throughout the day on most days. Some of her negative cognitions are related to feeling different than others and sometimes being too hard on herself about what she does or does not accomplish. She has never taken medication for mood stabilization but is open to considering the possibility.

Social: During the initial assessment she shares that she has been dating a man for five years. She feels he is a good person and a good friend. They have a great deal in common and she believes he will be her long-term partner.

She enjoys her job as an elementary school teacher. She feels safe in the community she lives in but would prefer to live near a larger city in the future.

She speaks with her mother and father a couple times a week. She describes the relationship as somewhat formal. She has not continued in the Christian religious principles of her family and this has been a disappointment to her them. She has three older siblings. They are all married and have children. Lizette says that she cares for them but does not have close relationships with any of her siblings.

Cultural: Lizette identifies as Latinx. Her parents are both from Mexico and immigrated to the United States before Lizette was born. She experiences pride in her cultural identity and seeks to engage in her community and traditions as often as possible. She notes that the shared cultural identity of her partner brings comfort and joy to her; however, he is not a Spanish speaker. Sometimes that inability to dialogue in Spanish on a regular basis is associated with loss and sadness.

Spiritual: She believes in a creator but feels a sense of confusion about her spiritual path because she no longer holds the beliefs of religion she was raised in or shared by her family. She notes a nagging feeling of guilt that has been present for quite some time in her life. She feels that religion played a role in this guilt so has tried to distance herself from the source.

Insert Diagnosis: Major Depressive Disorder, Mild

Many practitioners would feel enough information had been gathered about symptoms and domains of functioning up to this point and create an intervention plan. Providing assessment surrounding the domains of sexuality and intimacy would yield a much more expansive understanding of Lizette's life experience and symptoms.

Sexuality: Client reports feeling uncertain about how she identifies her orientation. She shares that the way that sexuality was depicted to her by her family and culture felt limiting and foreign to her. She feels embarrassed about some of the thoughts she has that make her excited and they feel extremely different from anything she does with her partner. She notes that ideas of domination in sex feel exciting, but she is confused if that means something is wrong with her.

Sexual Health/Intimacy: When asked about sexual needs and pleasure, Lizette shares that she is unaware of her needs and does not experience pleasure. She shares that she relies on her partner to direct intimacy and does what he wants. She notes that there is intermittent pain in intercourse. Although she is not familiar with signs of arousal in her body/mind she notes that her body never feels any different than usual when they are intimate. With tears and apprehension, she shares that she has thoughts that are pleasurable about women but feels a sense of guilt and impossibility about pursuing the path of intimacy with a woman. She notes that confusion and guilt surround intimacy. She describes feeling emotionally numb during experiences of intimacy as a way she "gets through it." The intimate experiences of Lizette and her partner are limited to intercourse with little foreplay. There is a great discomfort around him touching her genitals, and she has little interest in exploring other types of sexual play with him. She expresses that she has limited knowledge of health and pleasure, beyond use of condoms.

When a mental health professional opens the conversation of sexuality and intimacy with Lizette, the symptoms of depression take on a different meaning. Lizette is facing a great deal of confusion about her own sexuality and she has thus far lived in environments and relationships, which have dictated how to be, versus offering opportunity for exploration. Her fantasies related to intimacy with women are confusing and guilt-ridden. The routine of weekly intimacy with her partner requires emotional numbness and sometimes physical pain.

It is crucial to understand that if a mental health professional did not ask Lizette about her sexuality and intimacy, she would not share this information. In the same way that some mental health providers feel that it is inappropriate to discuss sexual health and sexuality, many clients also feel they shouldn't bring it up. Guilt, uncertainty, secrets, pain, and unexpressed desires are often unspoken and carried with clients through many years of their life. There is also the unspoken acknowledgement that these issues are not valuable if they are not worth asking about. Consent to discuss and acknowledgement of their importance are extremely important elements in introducing the topic of sexuality, sexual health, and intimacy.

When sexuality, sexual health and intimacy are skipped topics, glossed over or hesitantly mentioned, the vast majority of our clients will not ask for assistance or bring up concerns. The tone of voice and language used by the professional during an assessment signals comfort or discomfort. In addition, stigma, and oppression often limit what an individual considers as possible for themselves. They may not have words or ideas related to their sexuality, health, intimacy unless we can provide those words and space. The sexual health assessment will be explored in detail in Chapter 5 of this text.

Why the Silence?

Both medical and mental health professionals in the United States largely agree with the definitions of sexual health and sexuality set forth by The World Health Organization. Unfortunately, the majority fail to put into practice inclusivity of sexuality and sexual health in their basic assessment and intervention protocols.

Data reflects that for many providers of mental and medical health, the fear of offending a patient or not having answers to their questions are primary reasons professionals avoid the topic. There is also the issue of bystander effect paired with discomfort. When professionals do not feel comfortable or prepared to discuss the topic, they often report the belief that another professional or "expert" will address the issues, thus they do not need to.

Discomfort and concerns about professional boundaries are also cited. Practitioners have concerns that assessment questions may be seen as exploitative or crossing a professional boundary. A common concern of offending or causing discomfort to clients/patients is often cited in the medical and mental health professional community. This is more common when the gender of the client/patient is different from that of the practitioner (Quinn et al., 2011).

Access to Sex Therapy in the United States

Research repeatedly points to the lack of training as a prominent reason why mental health professionals do not discuss, assess or include topics of sex, sexuality, and intimacy. It is estimated that 80% of clients in psychotherapy settings are being seen for presenting problems related to sexuality. The vast majority of graduate-level programs for psychology, counseling, social work and therapy do not require any human sexuality courses. When they do require or offer the courses, it is most often focused on sexual health that includes topics like contraception and sexually transmitted infections (Burns et al., 2017; Nagoski, 2015).

When graduate education does not represent sexuality and intimacy as core curriculum it places this information as optional or "specialized." Post-graduate education certainly allows us to select areas on which we want to concentrate and learn even more. However, it is imperative that we complete our education with a basic understanding of how to discuss, assess, and treat concerns core to the human experience.

A very high percentage of our clients have experienced abuse and/or assault. We may learn how to gather the information about harm but most of our educational institutions do not offer coursework to address healing sexual selves and how to develop a sense of "intimate justice" in their lives. It would be a horrible injustice and cruelty to ask an individual if they experienced food scarcity on a regular basis and not offer any resources. The majority of social work and other mental health experts do exactly this related to the handling of sexual abuse and assault. This is a huge social injustice.

For professionals that believe they must have the resources to assess and treat sexuality, health, and intimacy, they often need to seek out specialized training because it is not provided in core curriculum. This is expensive and often out of reach for social workers. Advanced training in sex therapy requires 90 course hours in 15 topics of core areas of human sexuality from an accredited institution and an additional 50 hours of direct supervision. These are the requirements of The American Association of Sex Educators, Counselors, and Therapists (AASECT), the largest credentialing body for sex therapy certification (AASECT, 2022).

If we understand sex, sexuality, and intimacy to be a core element of the human experience, we cannot simply rely on the field of specialized providers or those with post-graduate training related to sex therapy to be the only practitioners that speak on these topics. To ensure that sexuality and intimacy can be competently addressed as a core component of mental health and well-being, we must ensure all mental health practitioners have access to training during their graduate education.

Continuation of Secrets

When we fail to discuss sexuality, we fail to capture critical information. The previous case example highlights how family history, experiences related to identity and current relational patterns intersect with sexuality in major ways. When we fail to explore sexuality we also take part in the continuation of shame and secret keeping surrounding this topic. In most cultural and religious experiences, in most societies, there is an unspoken rule that sex should not be discussed. Our silence on these topics are signals to our clients. "Can I ask you about sexuality?" is much different than "We've talked about lots of important areas of health, functioning, and identity and I would like to include sexuality in our conversation."

As you continue your journey through this text you will open yourself to exploration of what it means to enter into these topics, how to prepare yourself, how to have the conversations, what to listen for and how to help. This is justice work, imperative work, intentional work, necessary work. It is not optional but required.

Questions for Reflection and Discussion

Consider the setting of your placement or internship. Has your supervisor discussed incorporating sexual health into the interpersonal practice work? If so, how did this conversation feel for you? If not, how could you invite this topic into supervision?

Consider a client you have worked with or are currently working with in your internship. How might work change if sexual health and intimacy were introduced into the work?

Make Room for Yourself

2

My first assignment as a burgeoning sex therapist was to drive in my car and say, aloud, words like, climax, orgasm, vagina, penis, hard-on, erection, and dildo. . . . In weeks to come I would be sitting across from clients and asking them detailed questions about their genitals, their history of experience discovering their genitals, shame related to their sexual experiences, recent experiences of orgasms, erectile difficulty or vaginal pain. I needed to know not only what to say but how it felt within me to say these things aloud. I needed to know what it felt like to ask other individuals to talk with me about these things.

The stories, reactions, and emotions of the individuals seeking mental health services often seem to fill up the room. As a new clinician, I remember feeling sometimes exhilarated and at other times exhausted by the emotion and energy of a client session. Graduate courses failed to teach me how to make space for myself in that space. If we are going to use ourselves as a collaborative tool, we must have self-awareness, permission to share ourselves. Our reactions must be thoughtful, informed, and intentional. We need strategies to care for ourselves within that process. The added elements of sexuality and intimacy can often make this even more difficult for many mental health professionals, leading to fear and avoidance of the topics. This chapter will offer self-reflection strategies and tools to make room for your own emotions, attitudes, and experiences as you collaborate with clients.

Each of us lands somewhere on the comfort continuum regarding discussing sexuality. That comfort is based in generational influences, early

DOI: 10.4324/9781003166382-3

childhood messaging, peer influence, religion, and culture, exposure to messages and images, availability to sex education, your own experiences of body discovery, as well as relationships and sexual experiences. This is an opportunity to understand these influences and evaluate how you may want to challenge or expand your attitudes and comfort level related to these topics. Reflection can increase confidence and comfort as an individual and certainly influences relationships and parenting. Most important to the topic of this book, it is a necessary process as a mental health professional.

Activity/Reflection

The series of questions that follows reflects some of the questions that may be considered as part of a sex history timeline.

Part 1: Provide yourself a reflective space to consider these questions and write out the answers that come to mind. You may find this reflection to be a very emotional experience and benefit from taking some breaks and returning to the questions.

What was the first time you remember being aware of your own genitals?

Who do you remember asking questions to about your body? Were their responses helpful?

What was the first time you touched yourself and noticed pleasure?

What was the first time you masturbated?

What is a memory of having interest in touching another person's body related to interest/attraction?

Did you ever experience fear or shame related to feelings of attraction?

Do you recall any sexual play with peers as a child?

What is the first time you saw sex depicted in a movie or discussed in a text?

When was the first time you saw pornography?

Do you recall a time someone commented on your body as a child or adolescent?

Do you recall your awareness that your body was developing?

Do you remember comparing your body development to others?

(Foley et al., 2012)

Part 2: After responding to these questions in writing you can return to the material and use symbols or words to note the mood associated with the experiences. For example, symbols or words you might use as labels: happy, exciting, traumatizing, scary. Consider how these events influenced your feelings about your body, your sexuality, other people's sexuality. Consider how information/education and perhaps shame and fear were part of these early experiences. Some of the experiences you are reflecting on may bring up a feeling of gratitude while others may be accompanied by grief or sense of loss. It is important to note that and allow yourself to have space to feel these emotions.

Part 3: Select a trusted person in your life you would like to share a few of these reflections with and begin the conversation. Important to this process is ensuring consent. Often when we begin our own journey of discovery and reflection, we feel a sense of openness and energy, and this is not always a space that others in our lives share. It is important that we (1) describe the conversation we would like to have (2) ask permission of the listener (3) invite them to ask questions or share their own experiences if that would be beneficial. *Note that it is important to consider what you need from sharing and identify that with your listener before beginning to share. When we provide direction from those listening and engaging with our story, we are much more likely to feel emotionally satisfied and supported. Often we do not consider what would feel beneficial before opening up and leave conversations related to important emotional topics feeling unheard, lacking validation or overwhelmed by the response of the other. An example: "I'd really like to share some information I discovered about realizations about my body as a child and some of my mother's reactions. This information is pretty emotional so if you would be able to listen to my full story and then ask questions at the end it would be most helpful for me."

This exercise is invaluable in preparing you to listen to client stories as a mental health professional. It provides an experience of vulnerability. It is important to be aware that the questions we ask in intake material or during one-to-one sessions can be exciting, overwhelming, and often very upsetting for our clients. Preparation and support in the process, and of course never under-estimating the intensity of reflections such as these, is crucial.

This exercise also serves as preparation for assessing the values and bias you hold around topics of sexuality. Listening is an interactive process involving a host of explicit as well as implicit reactions. Too often, clinicians believe that they can pretend or avoid reactions unbeknownst to clients. We will discuss in Chapter 4 strategies to respond to clients as we become aware of our own emotions surfacing. The first part of that process is our own self-awareness of values and bias related to this topic.

Therapists trained in sex therapy participate in a Sexual Attitude Reassessment (SAR) experience. The SAR provides an opportunity to explore personal beliefs, attitudes, and bias related to a host of sexual experiences. The SAR often increases comfort with the wide variety of attitudes and practices and increases capacity to communicate about the diversity of sexual topics. Certainly, a written text cannot provide the experience of a SAR. The following exercise will provide an opportunity for reflection on your own values, beliefs, and attitudes.

Discovering Your Values, Bias, and Attitudes

The expansive landscape of sexual expression is beyond definition. Any object or experience has the potential to be erotic to a person. We often use our bodies to express our sexual desires and erotic expression yet it is in our minds that our erotic template, or core erotic theme, exists. Sexologist Jack Morin described the erotic template as "an internal blueprint for arousal. . . with recurring patterns" that often has little to do with love. Like most things, our society is not subtle in its suggestions of what is expected or ideal in the erotic, just as our society provides a limited scope related to body type, relationship type, etc. A good place to start in assessment of sexual values, attitudes, and bias is to recognize how limiting the assumptions we are fed by our culture can be. Understanding how these limitations have impacted you as an individual, helps you to welcoming more open and expansive perspectives. (Morin, 1995)

A rule you may have heard, "don't yuck my yum," is often a simple starting point I suggest when working with clients to communicate about erotic templates. Discussing, sometimes even acknowledging to yourself, what is erotic can be very vulnerable and scary. It is very damaging when judgement is the response to communication of your sexual fantasies and excitement. This brief exercise is a wonderful way to start welcoming in curiosity:

Activity/Reflection

Exploring and Sharing Your Erotic Template

Begin by allowing yourself a quiet space for reflection. Close your eyes if you feel comfortable and consider a fantasy that you have never shared with someone else. Don't be overwhelmed with the word fantasy. This does not mean it needs to be a detailed image or experience. A fantasy may be as simple as an image of a person or body part, an image or memory of your own body being touched in a certain way. A fantasy may even be something that you witnessed, or wish to witness, that does not seem to be sexual in any way, but it makes you excited/aroused when you think about it.

> Allow yourself to simply hold this image.
>
> Notice how your body feels. Is there a stirring in your stomach, warmth in your cheeks, perhaps sensation in your genitals?
>
> Imagine sharing this fantasy with another person.
>
> What words arise when you consider sharing your fantasy? Is there excitement, fear, worry or confidence associated with this idea?
>
> Now consider how you would want someone to respond if you shared this fantasy. Do you have any fears that their response might be different than what you wish? What influences this thought?

Hopefully this exercise provides some insight into the vulnerability related to sharing what is sexually exciting. It may also open your awareness into the shame that is often associated with our own erotic templates. Beginning by simply allowing, being curious, and not judging our own erotic template is a wonderful place to start. At risk of over-simplifying our own complexity, it is interesting to consider how we do not judge, question or hypothesize about sensations around taste and preference. When we enjoy spicy foods, tart, sweet or the combination, we generally are able to simply allow that as our preference. How we indulge may come with judgement or negotiation but simply allowing it to be our preference generally comes easily. The same can apply to our erotic template.

Activity/Reflection

Communication Regarding Erotic Template

> To expand this exercise, I ask you to place yourself in the space of receiver of someone else's information about the erotic.
>
> Give yourself a quiet place of reflection. Have a pen/paper handy to make some notes. Close your eyes if you are comfortable.

Imagine learning from a friend, coworker, neighbor a bit about their sexual excitement or fantasies.

Imagine the person sharing something that might be unexpected. Select one of these examples or create your own example.

Someone shares with you the experience of feeling aroused when being humiliated by another.

Or

They feel aroused by images of others being hurt.

Or

They feel excited about sexual play with feces.

What words come to mind when you imagine hearing this information?

Are there cognitions representing fear or judgement?

What sensations are you aware of in your body?

How would you like to respond?

What nonverbal expressions might be shared?

Are there aspects of your feelings that you feel you would have to hide or hold back to protect the sharer?

Self-Awareness and Authenticity

A great deal of our graduate training is focused on assessment and intervention. We need to know what to ask and what to say in response. In the field of social work, a great deal of attention is also placed in the collaborative relationship. We use this term so often, perhaps we don't always slow down enough to consider what it means or what it requires. True collaboration requires insight not just into the other, your client, but the awareness of what is occurring internally. This dance of awareness I believe is best described by the term mindsight, defined by Daniel Siegal. Mindsight helps an individual to see their mind and to shape it in a different way, towards health. The mind that we are shaping defined in this context as "embodied and relational process that regulates the flow of energy and information" (Siegal, 2010).

When we look internally, we train our awareness toward our emotional and somatic experience. This can be described as the "me map." For those of us that grew up with caregivers that were intentional and curious about helping us name and know our internal world through reflective dialogue, this work is likely automatically occurring throughout most moments. For those of us that did not have that early experience, we may need to be more intentional in developing this awareness. With a "me map" we are more capable of seeing the "you map" of the person in our context. This "you map" is what we sense or imagine they may be internally experiencing. This is crucial to the mindsight of the collaborative experience or the "we map" (Siegal, 2010).

The practice of tapping into our own internal experiences during our work with clients is imperative in responding with authenticity. As new practitioners it is common to feel distracted by formulating a response to the client's communication and losing track of one's own emotional experience in the moment. This is rarely discussed in most graduate programs; however, it is perhaps one of the most important elements of clinical work. The majority of knowledge gathered in our interactions with clients is implicit, depending on facial expressions, body posture, and tone of voice. Even when we are prepared to *say* the *right* thing the lack of insight or regulation of our internal experience may deliver a much different message.

Giving ourselves permission to have our own emotions is important. When we "make space for our emotions," we work to notice them and respond with compassion, rather than attempting to shut them down or push them away. The exercises that have been offered in this chapter assist in noticing specific thoughts as well as physical sensations related to sexual content. When we become familiar with the feelings, we can rather quickly notice the sensations while at the same time being present with another, as described in the definition of mindsight. Understanding our own history related to our sexuality allows us to respond to cognitions and sensations with compassion. A metaphorical nod to the feeling that has been raised that acknowledges, "I know this emotion or sensation and understand why it is popping up now" is an example of practicing this compassion with ourselves.

Cultivating our ability to practice mindsight can happen during our inter-actions outside of the clinical space. In fact, practicing this in our daily encounters with intention will improve communication and relationships throughout our lives. It can be useful to practice aloud, noticing, and providing compassion first, then moving to internalize the process. Verbalizing our internal process is not harmful even in a clinical space.

Activity/Reflection

"Noticing" Phrases With Clients

Sit across from another individual, ideally another student.

One person can offer a simple story related to a conflict with someone or a difficult encounter or emotion they experienced. This can be brief.

Practice using one of the following phrases in response:

When you shared that story, I felt. . .

I noticed (insert physical sensation) when you shared that story.

I need to pause and process my emotions as I share your story.

Discuss with your partner how this response felt for them.

Would you feel comfortable using this with a client? Why/why not?

The application of Polyvagal Theory in interpersonal practice work encourages this sharing of information to assist clients in self-regulation and interpersonal regulation. One way to utilize Polyvagal Theory is creating a map of the autonomic nervous system with clients so that they may be empowered to regulate and direct their states of being. We can also share our maps of the autonomic nervous system and then reference them as we work collaboratively. If I find myself in a sympathetic or more hyper-aroused state during a session with a client, I might share, "I'm noticing a shallowness to my breathing and wondering how your [the client] description of this trauma might have influenced me. Can you check in with what you are noticing in your [client] system? New practitioners can benefit from sharing their own experiences and also giving themselves permission to not have the right response or answers (Dana, 2020).

Engagement With Clients

Now that we have explored several ideas related to personal awareness in clinical settings it is important to consider how we offer comfort and curiosity to clients specific to conversations around sexuality.

"During our assessment I have asked lots of questions about your family history, profession, and educational history as well as mental health experiences. Your sexual health is also a key part of your well-being and I have several questions to ask about this as well." In the other domains of functioning, we proceed with interest rather than requesting permission. It is important that we normalize sexuality by incorporating it into the biopsychosocial assessment versus asking permission to include it as an add-on to our assessment.

For many clients, the communication you offer about their sexual selves may be the first engaging and positive conversation on the topic in their lifetime. It can be overwhelming, sometimes painful and scary, sometimes exciting and insightful. Our goal is to ensure that we begin by creating a framework for the conversation, that the process is consensual and empowering and the information is useful and informative.

Guidelines for Sexuality Assessment

> **Step 1**: Creating a framework: *Address purpose of gathering information related to sexuality *Explore history of past information-seeking or information-sharing related to sexual self
>
> **Step 2**: Ensuring consensual and empowering process *Consistently provide opportunities for client to express consent in process *Allow client to guide pacing of process
>
> **Step 3**: Purposeful and informative

Step 1: Introducing the Topic

Providing information about why we are asking about information about sexuality is very important because we are entering a topic that family, religion, and society have often deemed unspeakable. Therefore, we break a societal norm when we enter into the discussion with a client and need to clarify our purpose. Addressing these societal norms directly for clients can be very helpful. Inviting clients to assess what messages they received about communication about sexuality and how people responded to them when they attempted to ask questions can be a useful space to begin. Much like exploring issues of attachment or emotional neglect with clients, messages, and communication about sexuality is more often about what did not take place, what wasn't, rather than what was. This can be difficult for clients to identify what was painful or how they learned not to discuss this, without a comparison to what might have been. Sometimes questions that can guide clients in this exploration. You can contemplate these questions related to your own experience before trying them with clients:

Do you remember asking questions about your body parts to a family member or older adult? What do you remember about their response? Is there any implicit knowledge you gathered from their response?

Do you remember if there were messages about sexuality or sexual behavior in religious text or services during your childhood? Were they positive or negative? Did they create fear or shame when you received them?

Do you remember any conversations with peers sharing information about sexuality? What is the feeling associated with this memory? Do you know if the information was accurate or inaccurate?

Step 2: Creating a Consensual and Empowering Process

The topic of sexuality often comes with "BIG T" Trauma for many individuals. Unfortunately, most individuals identify "small t" trauma. In this context BIG T trauma may be sexual abuse, sexual assault, discrimination related to sexual orientation (this list is not exhaustive) and examples of "little t" trauma may include being shamed when asking questions about sex or receiving sex negative messaging from a religious institution. Using straightforward tools of permission and pacing, we can create a healing experience through our engagement in the assessment process.

Asking permission throughout the assessment process allows for the practice of consent.

> "I'd like to ask you about. . . (ex: your first sexual experience of being touched by another person sexually)?"
>
> "Do you feel comfortable moving forward with some questions about. . . (ex: your sexual orientation)?"
>
> "What is coming up for you as you discuss this topic?"
>
> "Does it feel safe and healthy to continue discussing this topic?"

When we are negotiating consent, we should ensure individuals feel open to choose to share or not share, can change their mind, understand what we are discussing and why we are discussing it.

We can help our clients by being very intentional about the process and helping them notice how it feels for them. The therapeutic relationship provides a space to experience a new way of being in relation to others and in relation to certain topics about ourselves. The experience of the sexual health assessment can offer healing as well as helping clients experience a new, positive way of engaging in the topic.

Let's look at these steps in the process in a brief example:

Therapist: (*Step 1: Introducing the topic*) Christie, I'd like to ask you some questions about your sexuality and your sexual health history. Sexuality is a very important part of our lives and many people don't have the opportunity to discuss and think about this aspect of themselves. Talking about this will help us understand your history and relationships in a fuller way. (*Step 2: Providing opportunity for client to offer consent*): Can we discuss some of the questions now?

Client: Yep, sure you are in charge.

Therapist: I realize so many doctors, specialists, etc. might have felt very much in charge of the process but I want to make sure you are in charge of how and what we discuss and how it feels to you. I'm going to check in often so we can notice how you are feeling together.

Client: Sounds good. I feel comfortable talking about this stuff here because you don't seem judgy.

Therapist   (*Step 2: Allow client to guide pacing of process*): I'm glad it feels comfortable right now. If that changes we can certainly listen to that. I am hearing that judgement has been a part of earlier experiences of talking about sexuality. I want to check in to make sure that isn't coming up now as we talk.

Client: Well. . . for sure. When I have told people that I had cervical cancer you can just see their face change. Everyone from my mom to doctors, talking about medical history sort of pause and think about me different.

Therapist: (*Step 3: Purposeful and Informative*): I am so glad you are sharing this. A medical experience that was likely scary and at times painful was something you have been judged for in the past. It is really important that you shared this with me because part of therapy is not only understanding how these major life experiences have shaped us, but also allowing space for expressing and getting in touch with emotions you may not have had permission or opportunity to feel. Many cancer survivors need space and time for grief and loss.

Client: Tears cover her face. I just felt like I had to shut my mouth and get through it because the way I got the cancer was considered my fault. I do need space just to feel all the stuff that came up during that time.

This example illustrates how the steps of engagement are embedded in our collaborative communication with clients. Reminding ourselves that it is the process, not simply getting answers to our questions, that is imperative. Listening for the patterns and themes that are addressed during this process helps us consistently connect the information to the larger intervention planning for the client. When we are grounded in the framework of engagement, we create a safe space that often allows for openness and flow as we explore the sexual health assessment.

For many readers, you have already begun your training of thinking on your feet. You have experienced that it is impossible to predict the content of any client session. The topics and content related to sexuality are quite expansive and we must be prepared for a terrific variety of terminology, presenting challenges, specific goals. Familiarity with common terminology and presenting topics related to sexuality, health, and intimacy is helpful.

Familiarizing yourself with terminology and concepts that feel foreign is a good way to be prepared to navigate and orient yourself. When we ask our clients questions, they have an expectation that we will be familiar with their world and their terms. We cannot know everything but keeping informed through podcasts, journals, and books, as well as having sources of reference in our network is very important. I would recommend owning your own copy of:

Handbook related to mental health medications

Human sexuality course book

Workbooks related to:

- Gender
- Sexual Health
- Mindfulness

Your journey through the activities and reflections of this chapter will hopefully help you feel more capable of navigating the moments of the unknown. Remember, authenticity, and mindsight help us remain curious and collaborative with the new and sometimes challenging content our clients have been invited to explore.

Questions for Reflection and Discussion

When you reflect on the activities in this chapter, which one was the most challenging for you? What did you learn about yourself through the exercise?

What are ways we can challenge bias from other professionals in the field?

Introducing Topics With Teenagers and Families **3**

Boundaries and Ethical Considerations

Introduction

Navigating conversations about sexuality can be complicated. Mental health professionals are often in a terrific position to have these conversations but lack the language and content that is developmentally appropriate. Concerns about boundaries and ethics are prominent concerns related to family values surrounding sexual health content.

Differentiating Sexual Values and Sexual Health

I realize that mental health professionals reading this book will be practicing in a diversity of communities and settings. Rural, urban, religious, agnostic, varying economic, cultural, and political identities will be held by your clients. It can feel frightening and sometimes paralyzing to open a topic with individuals that may be viewed as wrong, harmful or inappropriate. This is especially challenging when working with children and youth.

Experimentation, curiosity, and questioning are tools of differentiation, an important task of emotional and psychological development. Cultures and religions place differing values on the importance of differentiation, individuation or assimilation and dependence. From a practice of cultural humility, we should validate the values and norms of our client's cultural beliefs and practices. We can also help them to explore the difficulties, or pull

DOI: 10.4324/9781003166382-4

they may be experiencing, facing differing messages and values held by their particular culture and/or religion, and those of the dominant United States values and norms.

We do our best work when we define our roles with the agencies we work for, the supervisors we answer to, and the parents/caregivers that accompany youth to treatment. I describe my work as providing information about a person's body and health that can offer them the highest level of information for keeping themselves safe and healthy in their decision-making. I describe this as sexual health. I empower families/caregivers to be part of their child's journey by providing sexual values that they uphold.

An important rule to guide your work is to open the topic of sexual health with young people and to inform stakeholders of the basis of your information. I usually provide a metaphor outside the scope of sexuality such as nutrition. If I am discussing care for one's body and discussing nutrition, I might describe balance, portions, and types of food, including types of food that can be harmful in excess. I would certainly expect that the family would share values surrounding food that relate to religious requirements or cultural purposes of food related to traditions, joining or celebrating. We can imagine how these messages may be contradictory for the young person receiving health information and value information. Perhaps turning down food is considered disrespectful in their family/culture; however, they have learned about how excess red meat is not helpful to your body. Making sense of the varying messages and values from family, culture, and larger society is confusing. It is a developmental task of adolescence and young adulthood. It is not a reason to keep information from young people. It is important to deliver information that is developmentally appropriate and to offer space to discern the information and contradictions.

When a question exists, it is always important to provide an accurate answer. The level of detail may be determined by the developmental stage. Answers from parents or any caring adult that shut down or shame, such as "you shouldn't ask that, you're too young," for example, are simply harmful. They force young people to find sources other than their trusted people for answers and decrease the potential that we can help them with future decisions. An important rule for your work is to answer existing questions. When questions seem beyond the expected information that would/should be available to a child/adolescent, we might assume that something in their context has provided additional exposure to information. Since they cannot turn back the clocks and ignore that exposure, we should still give them the information they are seeking and also ask about how they have learned the information.

Developmentally Appropriate Sexual Health Material

As a mental health provider and social worker, I work from the belief that most children/youth are not receiving adequate information about their bodies, sexuality or relationships. Working from a social justice framework, part of my work is giving people access, permission, and opportunity to know themselves fully and be seen and be recognized by others in all their identities. The biopsychosocial framework of assessment (that guides the development of our interventions) includes:

Medical health/resources/history

Relational health/history

Environmental health/living situation/Risk-protective factors/ current/history

Work/financial health/resources/current/history

Mental health/protective-risk factors/prior symptoms and diagnosis

Lifestyle health factors/substance use/exercise/nutrition/sleep/ socializing/stress management

Sexual Health that includes several components:

Sexuality: A core experience of being human and who you are as a sexual being

Defined by SIECUS (Sexuality Information Education Council of the United States):

Sexuality encompasses the sexual knowledge, beliefs, attitudes, values, and behaviors of individuals. Its various dimensions include the anatomy, physiology, and biochemistry of the sexual response system; identity, orientation, roles, and personality; and thoughts, feelings, and relationships. The expression of sexuality is influenced by ethical, spiritual, cultural, and moral concerns.

(Sexuality Information and Education
Council of the United States, 2004)

Sexual Identity:

> Sexual identity is the sense of who one is as a sexual being and is fundamental human experience comprised of a person's sex orientation and sex-role.
>
> (Peterson et al., 2016)

Sexual Expression:

> Sexual expression is the manifestation of your sexual self through your sexual thoughts, sexual feelings and sexual behaviors; all of which are significantly mediated by bioculturally bound modifiers.
>
> (Peterson et al., 2016)

Most people have not been provided with safe spaces to ask questions. It is not enough to help people avoid injury or disease. Individuals deserve the opportunity to explore the many facets of their sexuality and how it influences other areas of functioning. Dimensions of sexuality can be considered in these primary domains:

> **Sexual self-satisfaction**: sexual health literacy, self-love, self-pleasure, access to sexual health care
>
> **Relational sexual satisfaction**: love toward others, sexual activity with others, social, and spiritual sexual acceptance
>
> **Medical sexual satisfaction**: sexual disease status, sexual hormone status, sexual pain status, sexual injury status, sexual reproductive status, sexual compulsivity status
>
> **Sexual identity satisfaction**: gender orientation, sexual orientation, sex-role orientation
>
> (Peterson et al., 2016)

It is possible to learn, teach, and explore these topics from birth forward. Consider the example of four- and five-year-old children gathering for story time. Some children will want to sit closely and touch often, others will feel a need for some distance. Embracing the teachable moment, we can help children learn and grow by helping them think about:

> How they are feeling? What do they feel in their bodies? What feels good to them about being near their friends? What parts of their bodies make them feel proud? (self-satisfaction)

What feels good about being close to other kids? How does it feel to be touched and what they enjoy (examples like holding hands and hugging)? What feels too much? Practice asking permission for touch and closeness and setting boundaries. (relational-satisfaction)

These teachable moments have been developed into a sexual health curriculum in many forms. One example is Our Whole Lives (OWL) Curriculum developed by the Universalist Unitarian Church and United Church of Christ. It is a reliable resource that considers sexual health information from kindergarten through adulthood within the psycho-social developmental needs and milestones. OWL provides content with the idea that "well-informed youth and young adults make better, healthier decisions about sexuality than those without complete information" (Wilson, 2014).

The Purpose of Pleasure

As mentioned in the introduction of this text, I found myself navigating hundreds of conversations about sexual abuse, assault, and trauma without any language or tools to guide healing. Becoming a sex therapist provided that language and those tools. I think it is very possible to simplify by considering how we ask about and guide clients toward pleasure. Author and researcher Peggy Orenstein considers the honest conversation about sexual pleasure in this way, "if we truly want young people to engage safely, ethically, and enjoyably we have to discuss what happens after yes [consent]" and this includes discussing the "capacity and entitlement to sexual pleasure" (Orenstein, 2016). In all domains of functioning the ideal we are working toward is a sense of enjoyment, pleasure, and wellness whether that is expressed in mood, work life, and living context. We often begin our work with clients at a foundational level of maintaining emotional, physical, and sexual safety. We use resources to build into an awareness of and expression of pleasure as we move upward from the foundational work.

Let's Take a Closer Look at the Process Through Nadia's Story

Nadia entered therapy begrudgingly per their mom and dad's "request." The presenting concern was Nadia's "attitude" and constant arguing with and rebelling against parental rules and cultural norms. Nadia was the first generation in their family born in the United States. Their parents immigrated from Lebanon and maintaining their connection to their cultural roots was very important to the family.

During our initial sessions we explored sexuality. Nadia didn't have much language around sexual identity and appreciated the permission to define themselves outside the box of their family, culture, and peers.

Social Worker (SW):	We have discussed a lot about your family, peers, and emotional health. I'd like to explore issues related to your sexuality and sexual health.
Nadia:	Yep. Like how my parents want to see me or how I actually am? I mean, are you going to try to fix me so I please them?
SW:	I'd love to know more about how you actually experience yourself. In terms of your parents, confidentially protects your information. Just to remind you, unless your life or others' lives are in direct risk, I will keep all your information confidential.
Nadia:	I mean, I don't know what is up with me. Not sure if I'm bi or pan or whatever! I mean, I watch all this different porn and a lot of it is hot so I'm so confused. Definitely, I know, I'm not like the girls at my school. For sure!
SW:	So, it sounds like you have some solid ideas about what you don't feel like or enjoy and are open to exploring.

While mom and dad used the pronoun *she*, Nadia realized that *she* was alright, but *they* really felt better. Nadia felt uncomfortable with what they defined as traditional feminine expression. They used words like tough, sturdy, and edgy to describe themselves when they felt attractive or sexy. The makeup, long hair, and nails their mother enjoyed really didn't fit Nadia. Nadia preferred unshaved legs and combat boots. They shared that they could imagine kissing some girls at school and some boys but not the boys at school. They would prefer the "softer boys, gentler, that would let them be move like the dude."

SW:	It seems like you definitely have your own style and way of expressing who you are.
Nadia:	Yep, super different from my mom. I know she wishes I was more like her. She still wants me to go get my nails done and straighten my hair. I don't care about that junk!

SW: What do you prefer?

Nadia: I mean, I just hate the femme stuff. I like things that make me feel solid, hard. It isn't really manly but it isn't girly either. I don't know. . . it is complicated.

SW: I really appreciate your insight. It sounds like this is about your gender identity and maybe also gender expression and sexual orientation.

As Nadia found a place to begin exploring themselves and feeling seen in the context of therapy, a lot of the argumentative behavior decreased. As trust quickly developed in the therapeutic context Nadia shared some of the confusion they felt about things that they felt were sexually interesting. They liked the idea of giving oral sex to girls and worried that it would be found out by family. They started to talk with a girl from their school and navigate interest and consent. During this same time, they decided to date a boy from the school as a cover, to not be discovered with an interest in girls. While becoming very excited about sexual expression with the girl from their school, Nadia also sought advice about anal sex. They wanted to keep the boy they were dating happy but didn't want to have vaginal penetration.

Nadia: Everything has just been so wild and confusing lately. I mean it has been cool.

SW: Tell me about what has been cool.

Nadia: Well, there's a girl. Don't forget you can't tell anyone. She's at my school. She's hot. Maybe that means I'm bi, queer, what the hell. . . I don't know. [Smiling and excited]

SW: Wow, you seem really happy. That's exciting.

Nadia: Well, until I get caught. I can't be with a girl. I got a cover though. This boy, he's alright, we are dating now.

SW: Do you want to date him?

Nadia: He's fine. He's not what I want but he distracts my parents.

SW: So how do you manage all of this?

Nadia: He and I go out. My mom is happy. I kiss him. He is happy. I sneak to see my girl, we are happy.

SW: Got it. If you didn't have to date this boy you wouldn't ?

Nadia: Oh, hell no!

The following steps were used to help Nadia navigate their experience. These steps do not need to be followed chronologically except for Step 1.

Step 1: Acknowledgement of Sexuality as a Domain of Functioning and Opening Up the Conversation

Identifying with parents/guardians of minors your role related to privacy, confidentiality, and health and education

For example, in dialogue with parents/guardians: "my role in your child's life is to provide advocacy, education, and guide exploration of ideas in every domain of life. That includes many topics related to sexuality. I will also provide information related to mental, emotional, physical, sexual health and well-being."

SW: I am grateful you have trusted me to help your child in navigating these challenges. I will give them information about their body and their health and I hope you will continue to provide information about values that guide them.

Step 2: Discussing Sexual Identity

When we discuss sexual identity, we are using a term that holds many identities within it or that exists to compose our full understanding of our sexual identity. These include:

1. Sex Orientation
   Male (having testicular/masculinized tissue present)
   Female (having ovarian/feminized tissue present)
   Intersex Transgender (having some combination of testicular and ovarian tissue present)
   Psychosocial Transgender (not intersex but having psychological gender identity differing from sex assigned at birth)
2. Sexual Orientation (aka Sexual Orientation Pattern to denote more fluidity)
   Gay
   Bisexual
   Straight
   Asexual
3. Sex-Role Orientation (aka Gender Role)
   Traditionally Masculine (high masculinity/low femininity)
   Traditionally Feminine (low masculinity/high femininity)

Androgynous (high masculinity/high femininity)
Undifferentiated (low masculinity/low femininity)

(Peterson et al., 2016)

An initial assessment can incorporate the following terms in the form of inquiry:

GENDER IDENTITY

How do you describe your gender identity or internal sense of gender? Do you understand gender as a continuum? What language do you use to describe your gender? Is it safe for you to use these pronouns and definitions in family, peer, and community spaces?

GENDER EXPRESSION/PRESENTATION

How do you express gender through clothing, hairstyle, voice, language, body movement, and shape? Do you feel a desire to express this differently? Do you feel interest in doing so but not permission or safety in expressing your gender as you would like to?

SEX ASSIGNED AT BIRTH

What was your sex assigned at birth? Does that align with your identity? Does it feel painful or difficult to discuss?

ORIENTATION/SEXUAL ATTRACTION TO OTHERS

What groups or genders of people do you find yourself sexually attracted to? Do you experience a lack of sexual attraction?

ROMANTIC/EMOTIONAL ATTRACTION TO OTHERS

What groups or genders of people do you find yourself romantically, emotionally or spiritually attracted to?

(Hoffman, 2017)

It is so important to approach the assessment material with collaborative curiosity. In general, I have found that younger clients are more able to embrace these questions with interest and less intimidation. An "othering" exists for many clients with the belief that these sorts of assessment questions are "just for gay or transgender people." As a clinician I maintain interest, educate about gender and orientation as necessary and remain grounded in the importance in these questions for all clients. It often opens a door for further curiosity and sometimes permission to bring up difficult experiences in their history or questions that can be addressed in sessions.

Identity Exploration is truly an integral part of being human and experienced across the lifespan. The people, places, and experiences we encounter influence our organic sense of ourselves. Fluidity related to gender, orientation, and sexual expression, and practice has existed throughout history. The language we use to define this and the socio-political responses often suppress exploration and understanding. Certainly, limitations of expressing and being seen and identified in our true selves is directly correlated with stigma and interferes with mental health and wellness. As mental health practitioners we can provide space for every individual to explore and increase their understanding of themselves. This should be baseline assessment work, not incorporated only because a client initiates the conversation. Additionally, our work may offer healing related to community, family, religious stigma, and oppression of their identities, as well as resources to offer validation and support lived experience of their identities.

This work is especially important with youth because they don't have the same access to external resources as adults. These resources in the form of community programs, educational resources, and online communities may be directly blocked by some families or the youth may not have the information or language to identify.

SW: I'm wondering if it might be interesting to explore some definitions together related to sexual identity?

Nadia: I'm game.

SW: It sounds like you feel like a girl but not in the way that your mom expresses being a woman?

Nadia: I don't think I'm trans or non-binary. I'm cool with those folx but I feel like a girl.

SW: I can tell you have thought about this a lot. Do you have friends that you are able to talk this through with?

Nadia: Not so much. I mean, some of my friends know that I'm bi. At least I'm pretty sure that's what I am. I could just never let my family know that.

SW: What do you fear about your family's reaction if they were to know you were bi?

Nadia: They would lecture me about it being against God. My mom would be so devastated. She would probably deep down, hate me.

SW: I'm noticing that you are able to separate the way your family feels about bisexuality from how you feel about yourself. Even though it is so difficult and maybe even lonely not to have their support, it is important that you are able to know that your identity is wonderful.

Step 3: Discussing Sexual Expression

Sexual expression is informed by sexual fantasies, imagined sexual experiences that bring erotic pleasure, sexual behavior, the sexual things we enjoy doing to bring sexual pleasure and mediators of sexual expression, such as age, SES. When working with young people we can recognize that they are in the beginning stages of learning about themselves in terms of sexual expression. The following information can be useful to explore with clients to develop a working understanding of sexual expression:

- Identify current sources of information that influence the client's idea of about "how to be sexual." This may include:
  - School (sex education classes)
  - Religious/Community (youth group, LGBTQIA+ groups, scouting)
  - Parents, cousins, siblings
  - Pornography
  - Medical professionals

As you discuss these sources important considerations for the client: Do messages from sources contradict? Are they limiting, heteronormative, stigmatizing? Are they inaccurate?

- We develop an understanding of pleasure and preference for sexual behaviors through independent sexual discovery as well as interpersonal sexual discovery. It is important to understand how youth have access to this discovery and how they feel about exploration. Discuss resources for personal and relational learning:

Is there access to privacy for exploring one's own body or being sexual with other people?

Are there rules against self-discovery and masturbation in family, culture, community, religion?

Does the individual good about self-discovery and masturbation?

Do friends communicate about sexual expression in consensual ways?

- Identifying values that guide sexual behavior:

Does the individual listen to or receive messages from their body (pain, arousal, fear sensation)?

Does the individual have adults, peers or leaders in their life that they admire and take advice from related to sexual behavior?

Has the individual had experiences of trusting their decisions and setting boundaries related to sexual behavior?

- Identifying, creating or modifying sexual decision making:

Discuss a recent experience making a sexual decision (examples might include whether to touch themselves in a pleasurable way or whether to share a sexy picture of themselves).

Use this example to explore:

Were there ideas about pleasure or performance that they considered?

Did they imagine any risks/benefits to behavior?

Was there fear of doing or not doing the behavior?

Did it turn out well?

What were the repercussions or benefits afterwards?

**As we explore these questions, the clinician is listening for levels of autonomy in decision-making, degree of self/other pleasing, and shame/fear involved in decision making. This helps to consider ways we can increase or modify the decision-making process to improve outcomes.

- Defining goals

When we gather information, we are able to identify areas for development, healing, and change. As you summarize the information shared, work to recognize with the client that sexuality is influenced, and influences the other domains of functioning in a variety of ways. Defining goals related to sexuality may certainly influence relationship patterns, social anxiety, self-confidence. Work to identify specific goals related to:

- Increasing access
- Increasing information
- Comfort and acceptance of self
- Curiosity and self-discovery
- Establishing resources

SW: You seem really clear about your sexual orientation and also your gender expression. What are some people or places that have helped you to learn about this?

Nadia: Not school, not family, mostly not friends. The internet. Porn.

SW: So you have done a lot of work all on your own to figure yourself out. What kind of sources on the Internet have been helpful?

Nadia: I mean, there isn't one site in particular. Just learning about terminology and reading about other people's stories. It helped just to know that there are people out there like me. And as I move up in school, there are a few more people that are kind of out, quietly out.

SW: Quietly out? Meaning out in some spaces with some people?

Nadia: Right, like there is a girl I like at school and a few people know that. But, I also am acting like I'm into this guy at school so the rest of the people at school think I'm into him.

Step 4: Exploring Pleasure Within Sexual Expression

Initially we want to cultivate an awareness of pleasure and what it feels like for the person. For many people, pleasure is limited, sometimes it happens but is not pursued, and it is not always known what brings pleasure.

How would you describe feeling pleasure? (relaxed, silly, energized)

What are activities that bring about pleasure in your life? (running, eating ice cream, walking a dog)

Do you feel pleasure alone and in connection with others?

Do you feel there is an adequate amount of pleasure in your life?

Once a client has a grasp on pleasure in a general way, we can move the awareness into pleasure in sexual expression.

Have you experienced sexual pleasure on your own?

Do you have any feelings about the ways you experience sexual pleasure?

Would you be able to describe to another person what brings you sexual pleasure?

When you are sexually involved with another person what feels most important to you?

Do you feel like other people you have been sexually involved with have been interested in your pleasure?

SW: You seem to be clear about what you like and what you don't like. Tell me a bit more about what feels good to you or what brings you pleasure?

Nadia: I mean, I like things that make me curious. If I'm learning and thinking, then I'm usually happy. I like being outside. I like laughing and just being silly.

SW: So, trying new things, learning about new things is fun and brings you pleasure. It also feels like there is a really relaxed, carefree part of you that just likes to have fun with people.

Nadia: For sure.

SW: Have you been able to discover that same part of you in your sexual expression?

Nadia: Well, not the silly part but the learning part. With Lena, the girl I like, I feel curious but I feel uncomfortable about trying stuff because I wonder if I am going to do it wrong. It isn't like when I am with the guy who likes me, he sort of takes the lead and I follow. With Lena, I feel like I should know what to do and I get scared I'll do it wrong.

SW: That makes sense that it can feel like a lot of pressure to do it "the right way." I wonder if Lena might feel some of the same ways? Do you feel like she is curious about what you are into or what brings you pleasure?

Nadia: Yep. She's kind of shy but I know she cares.

SW: Sometimes if you can focus on what you feel excited about and what you imagine bringing you pleasure, it can give you insight about what to explore with another person. Can you picture in your mind what would be exciting to do with Lena?

Nadia: I can imagine it.

SW: If you can add to that, ways you might describe that sexual experience to Lena, that might be great practice.

Step 5: Harm Reduction

What are all the risks involved in the sexual behavior that is being considered or being done on a regular basis? (Should include relational, psychological, emotional along with the medical and physical)

> What would be the consequence if the sexual behavior was avoided? Another way of asking: Why is the behavior important despite the risk?
>
> Can we consider ways to make the risk less severe? Another way of asking, Can we think about ways to make the behavior a little safer?
>
> Do you imagine this decision changing in the future?
>
> What would it take for this to change in the future?

SW: I know you mentioned that you are hanging out with a boy at school and he kind of takes the lead on stuff you do together. Can we talk a little about that?

Nadia: [Lets out a big sigh.] Well, we have mostly been kissing which is, fine, it's whatever. Sometimes I will give him a hand job. He keeps saying we should go further but I told him I don't want to get pregnant. So he said we could do butt sex.

SW: Is that something you are interested in doing?

Nadia: Not really. It seems an alright compromise I guess.

SW: Do you have any information about butt sex or anal sex?

Nadia: I mean, I think it might hurt. I'm not excited about that.

SW: So there is some worry about it. Are there risks to not having anal sex with him?

Nadia: Well, having him around keeps my family and people at school from wondering about me and Lena. If I keep putting him off, I worry he will get bored.

SW: That sounds like a lot of pressure. It can be harmful to do things that you don't feel interested in. Even if your body is protected it can be uncomfortable, scary, and sometimes traumatizing to do things sexually that we don't want to do.

Nadia: Yep, I guess. But I think I can just try it and get it over with.

SW: If you did decide to have anal sex there are some things that will keep you safer. Can I offer some information?

Harm Reduction as a Public Health Approach to Sexual Health

Harm Reduction was first recognized as a public health approach in the 1980s in the treatment of substance use disorders. It was recognized that because some populations were not able / interested in eliminating use, harm reduction was important. Substantial evidence points to morbidity and mortality decreases in the treatment of substance use disorders, as well as HIV other STDs and more recently with teen pregnancy and risky alcohol use (Bigler, 2005).

When using harm reduction as a therapeutic approach when working with teens and sexual health, it is important to recognize is an intentional choice not an avoidance of addressing an issue. If we simply don't discuss a concern with a client because we assume they are going to go about things a certain way, we aren't practicing a harm reduction approach, rather avoidance. In the case of Nadia, they seemed fairly adamant that they were going to have anal sex with the boy they were dating. The ineffective approach of abstinence-only would be to tell Nadia that it is wrong and harmful to do at their age and they should not do it. The ineffective approach of avoidance is often taken by clinicians who do not want to offend their clients or come across as judgmental.

The harm reduction approach requires we address behavior that has the potential for negative outcomes in a straightforward manner. We name the behavior and the potential negative consequence; for example, "I am concerned that having anal sex without any condoms or lubrication may hurt your body, cause emotional trauma or put you at high risk for an STI." We then are able to partner with our clients to brainstorm ways to reduce the risk.

So, What About Nadia?

In the first meeting with Nadia and their parents I discussed my role related to sexual health versus sexual values. I made space for sharing resources and education in a confidential framework. (Step 1: Acknowledgement of sexuality as a domain of functioning and opening up the conversation)

By the second session I was asking questions about sexual identity. Nadia appreciated being an expert of themselves. Therapy quickly became a space where they were seen in a way that they weren't seen in other domains of being. These initial conversations allowed Nadia to look more deeply into how they felt limited by their family and culture. A lot of pushing against their parents comes from this inner sense that the way they are isn't perceived as "right." Having a language for the ways that they are different in identity lead very easily into how they have come to learn about themselves, related to sexual expression. (Step 2: Discussing Sexual Identity)

Nadia spent much of their life feeling like "the other." They often pretended at school and found their own resources to explore sexual expression through pornography and on-line research. Dispelling myths, providing accurate information and expectations was important to help Nadia find ways to feel emotionally safe to begin exploring a relationship with a girl. The closer Nadia got to living out their own truth, the less anger and rebellion happened at home. As a therapist I needed to remember my role in helping Nadia navigate their journey and provide sexual health information versus values. We often talked about the risks of having peers or family find out about their gender or orientation identity. Nadia was open to discussing fears about "doing it wrong" related to oral sex with a girl. (Step 3: Discussing Sexual Expression)

Nadia certainly had given themselves permission for masturbation and this had allowed them to know themself. Communicating about their body with a partner felt uncomfortable and difficult and in session Nadia talked about words that felt more comfortable to use. Nadia was surrounded by friends and relationships in their family that focused on intimacy as an exchange versus intimacy for pleasure. It was important to think about that and what they wanted for themselves. The relationship with the boy from school fit that exchange framework and provided a sense of safety for Nadia. There was the worry of being defined as a lesbian in the community or by the family. There was also an internal confusion about how they felt about sexual expression with a girl. They were navigating the right to pleasure in the relationship with a girl and needed help navigating harm reduction in their relationship with the boy. (Step 4: Exploring Pleasure Within Sexual Expression)

I worried about Nadia in the sexual relationship with the boy from school. I worried how it would impact them emotionally and of course the concerns for anal tearing/injury or STIs related to anal sex. We talked about the cost/benefit of the relationship as well as why the anal sex felt necessary. I provided information about lubrication and anal sex. I discussed ways to introduce anal penetration on their own so they could better understand how it would feel and be more prepared. Nadia ended up having anal sex and really hated it. They didn't like the boy and felt sad about being in that situation with him. They ended the relationship with him and kept the relationship with the girl. They told their parents about their pronouns and that they liked girls but didn't talk about dating a girl. Their parents felt I had something to do with Nadia going down "the wrong path." We met several times as a family to work toward repair, increasing acceptance, and support. (Step 5: Harm Reduction)

Navigating Parental Resistance

There will be times that the assessment will yield alliance in identities and parental support. For many clients whose sex assigned at birth does not align with gender identity or expression there is often denial, resistance, anger, and sometimes emotional abuse/neglect or violence from parents and caregivers. This can be extremely difficult to navigate and it is recommended that ethical considerations on this topic can be explored in classroom conversations and in clinical supervision. A few points to guide ethical framework for these challenges:

Why does the parental/caregiver resistance exist? (fear for child's safety, transphobia or homophobia, lack of education regarding identify)

Is the child/youth emotionally safe and physically safe in current environment? What is the toll on mental health related to parental denial/resistance? Does the lack of support for transition/expression result in physical harm? (disordered eating, self-harm, lack of resources for binding, etc.)

Are there resources in the school, peer group, community that could increase support for the youth?

Are there figures of respect/support in the parent/caregiver's life/ community that could offer support in the process of addressing denial or resistance?

As clinicians we often feel intimidated by parents/caregivers who are dismissive of their child/youth's identity. It is imperative that we offer respect, support, and validation of name, pronouns, and other aspects of social identity. Framing respect for identity as aligning with emotional health and well-being of the child and youth allows us to navigate this space between parent's beliefs/wishes when they are in contradiction to their child's reality.

Parental resistance to sexual expression most often exists because of adults' own discomfort with the topic. Honesty and confidence in how you approach your work with children/youth is the very best way to manage parental/caregiver resistance related to sexuality. Having clear expectations and boundaries in our work models positive interaction for our clients and also helps all involved in the therapeutic relationship to feel safe.

We also use honesty and confidence to be very direct when we notice resistance early on in the therapy relationship. This may present in many forms, including clients chronically late to appointments, rushing therapy ("when will my child be better?") or a very guarded presentation related to the clinician. When we bring the issue up, we create an opportunity for underlying emotions/concerns to be investigated. Daniel Siegel, Clinical Professor of Psychiatry at the UCLA School of Medicine, uses a skill for repair and de-escalation called Name It to Tame It. I have found this simple tool extremely useful when working with adults as well.

Steps to Name It to Tame It:

1. Connect
   Both verbally and nonverbally, we can express care and welcoming. Ideas might include eye contact and statements such as "I'm really glad you made it here."
2. Name the emotion (you are taking a guess at the underlying emotion not the behavior being demonstrated)
   Examples might include, "I'm wondering if you are feeling scared for your child?" or "I'm wondering if you are feeling worried about where this conversation might lead?"
3. Offer of support/help
   Examples might include, "We can take it slow or you can ask for a break from the conversation at any time" or simply, "How can I be of support?"

(Siegal & Hartzell, 2003)

All of the material in this chapter could pertain to work with adults. Why is this chapter focused on children and adults? The first reason is that some special techniques are required to navigate sexual health terrain with children and in negotiation with their families. The second reason is that when we are able to start early in recognizing a person's sexual needs, identity, and worth, so much growth is possible and so much pain and negative consequence is avoided. Many of the adults we work with in the field of social work and mental health have been harmed by lack of resources, denial of their sexual identity, shame held about their sexual expression, and medical and physical damage due to a lack of safety. It is exciting to work with children and adults and be involved in helping them build a healthy relationship with themselves and a safe path in their world.

Questions for Reflection and Discussion

When you consider your own sexual health education, do you recall any acknowledgement of sexual pleasure discussed? How did the information influence your early experiences?

When reflecting on the case study about Nadia, what are some of the concerns that you feel about the case? Has your training or supervision encouraged you to address issues with teenagers in a different way than outlined in this chapter? Please describe.

What Could Go Wrong?

4

Introduction

Consider the places we traditionally talk about sex. Trading tales with friends, flirting, maybe discussing problems or concerns in a doctor's office. We often do not have opportunity to explore who we are as sexual people, what we struggle with, what excites us, who we want to be or how we express our sexuality. For 25 years of my career, I have welcomed these conversations. The primary reactions are very emotional. Tears, anger, surprise, and fear surfaces for many people. Helping clients separate out what these emotions mean for them is both healthy and ensures the emotions will not be projected onto us as clinicians. For instance, the client feeling shame about discussing a sexual preference might read the clinician's facial expression as distaste and comment, "you think that is gross, right?"

Framing the conversation is important, as is discussed in Chapter 3. Encouraging clients to identify the emotion associated with sharing information is also helpful. Sometimes that may require going a layer deeper than the surface response. While we don't want to insert our own emotions onto clients, it is helpful to consider the common emotions that are brought up surrounding this topic.

Uncovering the Feelings About the Feelings

The modality of Emotionally Focused Therapy, a blend of experiential therapy and attachment theory developed by Susan Johnson, investigates

DOI: 10.4324/9781003166382-5

primary and secondary emotions. Primary emotions are the initial emotional reactions to an event/discussion and secondary emotions are the feelings about the feelings. We help clients decrease guardedness and avoidance and increase emotional insight by exploring the secondary emotions. The secondary emotions often are reasons we project, reject or distance from the emotion or expression of the emotion (Johnson, 2019).

> **Initial Reaction**: Reflective/Interested
> **Underlying Emotion**: Curiosity
> **Underlying Emotion**: Confusion

> **Initial Reaction**: Defensive/Limited Insight
> **Primary Emotion**: Excited
> **Secondary Emotion**: Embarrassed

> **Initial Reaction**: Anger/Avoidance/Minimizing
> **Primary Emotion**: Shame
> **Secondary Emotion**: Fear

We explore these emotions with clients by noticing the initial reaction or behavior:

> "I notice you reacted with some pulling away or quieting down. What do you notice you are feeling as this occurs (this is the primary emotion)?" The client may answer, "it feels gross and shameful to think about doing that."
>
> The therapist then works to increase insight into secondary emotions, "shame and gross is a lot to experience. What reaction comes when you feel that?" The client may answer, "I don't know, I guess like a little kid and that is scary. . . fear."

The use of primary and secondary emotions identification can call attention to the underlying emotional experiences based in a lot of client attachment experience. It can also serve as a wonderful tool to investigate some of the common avoidance and reactive defensive strategies that can sometimes be overwhelming for new clinicians to address (Johnson, 2019).

Sexuality and intimacy are difficult topics for most clients. We should expect some difficulty and be prepared to offer collaborative investigation into what is coming up for clients. We should also be prepared to challenge the client. In Interpersonal Practice we consider these as affective constellations, the sequence of feelings. Two primary affect constellations are:

Anger-Sadness-Shame and

Sadness-Anger-Guilt

The first emotion is what generally presents for the client, either anger in constellation one or sadness in constellation two. That means that when you are exploring a relational topic the client will commonly express this emotion first. The second emotion in the constellation is what the client needs to be in touch with more and the third emotion is what the client will often feel when they do allow the second emotion. Confused? Here is an example of an affect constellation at work:

Therapist:	You shared that your partner often ends sex abruptly. Can you say more about that?
Client Brenda:	I work really hard to bring him pleasure through penetration and oral sex and I just feel sad. . . . Well it hurts my feelings when he just gets off and then leaves the room.
Therapist:	It sounds like you really put a lot of energy into his pleasure and when he leaves quickly that doesn't feel acknowledged.
Client Brenda:	Right, I mean not even saying anything, or even trying to bring me some pleasure! I mean I think I deserve that. It kind of makes me angry that he can be so selfish!
Therapist:	I'm really glad you are able to recognize that there is anger there too.
Client Brenda:	Well, I mean, maybe it isn't right to judge him. I mean I'm sure I'm not perfect either (There's the guilt).
Therapist:	It seems like when you allow yourself to feel the anger, it is hard to give yourself permission to stay there long. You felt guilty for feeling the anger. Why do you think that is?

In this example the therapist knows that Brenda is generally centered on the emotion of sadness and believes that it is beneficial for the client to bring awareness to the other emotions. The therapist also expects that guilt will arise when Brenda gets in touch with the generally unprocessed emotion of anger. It is expected because these affect constellations are common for many clients. Often the guilt or shame surfaces because of learned experiences of not being able to express necessary emotions. When we help clients get in touch with the lesser-expressed or never-expressed emotion, we truly help them make movement in insight and relationships. We can also save ourselves strife in the therapeutic relationship because the avoidance or projection of the emotions will not muddy the water of our relationship with the client (Teyber, 2017).

Permission to Discuss Sex

A common way for professionals to justify avoiding the discussion of sexuality with clients is to label the topic inappropriate, the work of someone else or unimportant. In our larger culture, talking about sex is often considered provocative and flirty. It is important for us to understand the value for ourselves and to share this. Talking about sex can change the world. By introducing the topic, I am helping individuals to end secrecy and shame, to explore important elements of their emotional and relational lives and to increase access to safety and wellness. It can be helpful to take a moment to consider your own values around sexuality and wellness.

Personal Insight Exercise

1. What is the cost to individuals when their sexuality is ignored, stigmatized or limited? List one or two words/phrases to describe that:
2. When you think about the therapy relationship, what do you hope to provide for your clients? List three words or phrases that describe it:
3. If you had someone who had given you resources, validation, and full acceptance related to your sexual identity and expression early in your life, how would you have felt? List three words that describe that feeling:

Hopefully this exercise provides some clarity and inspiration for what brings you to sexual health, mental health, and social justice work. You can use the words and phrases to help build what I call your elevator speech. Your elevator speech is a brief statement that describes why and how you do your work.

Use your first word/phrase of the reflection to lead your statement.

Your second words/phrases to describe how/what you do

Your third words/phrases to describe what is important or what is the outcome.

Here is my example of my elevator speech. I use this to advocate for the work at presentations or meeting people and describing my work. I use this to introduce the work to my clients:

Talking about sex can change the world. By introducing the topic, I am helping individuals to end secrecy and shame, *(this is the cost/what goes wrong)* to explore important elements of their emotional and relational lives *(what I will do/how I will do it)* and to increase access to safety and wellness. *(what is important or the outcome)*

While meeting with a new couple you open the conversation up to their history of intimacy. The wife frowns and then states, "do you think you are an expert on sex positions or something?"

What can you share from your elevator speech that might clarify your role/position?

A parent asks you if you are going to talk to their teenager about sex. "My daughter keeps trying to learn about sex and my husband and I think she's fast."

What can you share from your elevator speech that might clarify your role/position?

Considering Cultural Differences

We must also consider that sexuality is experienced through the lens of culture. A consistent driving force is wellness and access to information.

Objectively, condoms are a sexual safety tool that reduces the transmission of sexual infection and disease and reduces the risk of unwanted pregnancy. The use of condoms holds many meanings within cultural contexts. Some cultural messaging associates condoms with decreased "manliness" or sends a message of promiscuity if an individual wants a partner to use a condom.

Objectively vaginal lubrication serves a biological purpose, to protect tissues from fissures and decrease dryness. Some cultural messaging associates vaginal lubrication to promiscuity and "dirtiness."

As mental health professionals we seek to understand the values and beliefs that shape our clients from a cultural, community, family, and religious or spiritual aspect. During an initial assessment using a biopsychosocial framework a woman shared with me that her labia majora and labia minora (sometimes referred to as the lips of the vagina) as well as external clitoris had been removed. In the social/medical context of the United States this is often referred to as female genital mutilation. The safety of the therapeutic relationship allowed this individual to explore her feelings about this from a multi-cultural lens. As a Somali-American woman she held a feeling of protection toward her mother. Since immigrating to the United States, she noted that doctors, friends, and partners held judgement toward her mother, who elected to have this procedure completed when she was 11 years of age. She felt protective of her mother because in the community she lived in Somalia, having her labia and clitoris would have resulted in judgement and perhaps difficulty marrying. While her memory of the removal of her body parts was very traumatic, she also held deep compassion for her mother. Her experience living in the United States and partnering with an African American man, who was born and raised in the United States, also influenced her cultural experience of her body. The limitation of pleasure through sexual experience was something she was able to grieve with her partner.

We ground ourselves in clients' cultural context that influences their understanding of body, pleasure, and sexuality. When we allow the client to lead from their cultural experience, we can develop goals that are aligned with the client's cultural experience. Providing basic information about health fits nicely in this framework and allows the client the opportunity to incorporate the information into their context. For my client in the earlier example, the description of her experience from her multicultural lens allowed space for pride and understanding of her mother. She acknowledged her mother was acting out of protection and had experience of generational trauma. It allowed her to feel sadness and grief, to be respectful as a woman in her culture also required the loss of pleasure and risk of illness. It allowed feelings of hopefulness. Feeling understood and processing her experiences, she was able to consider health concerns related to her body, as well as new ways to introduce sexual pleasure into her life.

Blending Sexual Health, Social Justice, and Therapy

As social workers we are guided by the ethical principles of Social Justice and Dignity and Worth of the Person, as two of six ethical principles in the code of ethics. We hold the complexity of sharing sexual health information in a manner that is respectful of the identities held by each client we serve and their interpretation of health, wellness within the context of their religion, communities, and culture.

As mental health professionals, we explore identities and understand the client's definition of health and wellness through a collaborative framework and strength-based lens. The integration of sexual health, social work and social justice, and therapeutic practice is truly complex. Sexual health offers objective information related to the body and safety and objective measures of health. We use this to provide information in a way that offers choice and empowerment. Education and resources should always be utilized and paced based on client's situation and readiness to apply them. Exploring all the types of birth control available is not useful for a client whose religious beliefs condemn birth control.

Sometimes "what goes wrong" is that we over-educate, which can feel disempowering, overwhelming, and sometimes disrespectful. It can be exciting to share information that we believe will help our clients. When practicing consent in the interaction we should pay close attention to body language as well as verbal messaging. Paying attention to comfort and interest to the material can help us determine pace and how much to share.

PLISSIT

PLISSIT is a model developed by Jack Anon to help determine the differing level of intervention an individual client may need. PLISSIT stands for Permission Limited Information Specific Suggestions Intensive Therapy. The model works to ensure that mental health practitioners are intervening at the most basic level first. This model encourages the practitioner to be guided prominently by the client's comfort level and interest in engaging in specific interventions. We will discuss the guidance of PLISSIT in more detail in Chapter 11. I offer it as a reference and guiding principle. When we offer Limited Information as a sexual health resource, we are able to test if that small amount of information may be enough to meet the client where they are at and create *enough* change *necessary* for the client (Taylor & Davis, 2007).

Use of Language

Determining your stance on language is imperative as a mental health professional. The use of clinical language of our field can serve to be educational and provide a shared communication tool. It can also become distancing and serve to increase the inherent power dynamic between client and clinician. Using the client's language can feel either empowering or intrusive and belittling.

Take the example of a client that describes their emotional experience as "crappy." How have you been feeling in the past few days?" Response: "just real crappy." We work to first identify a shared understanding of the client's language. "Is crappy something you feel more in your body or your thoughts? . . . Does feeling crappy impact your sleep?" Once we gather more information about the definition, from the client's perspective, we must then determine if we continue using the client's language or transition to our clinical descriptions. We might also offer some education regarding symptoms and weave in clinical language.

Asking permission to use the client's language can incorporate a process of consent and respect: "It sounds like crappy is associated with a lot of the symptoms we see in what the diagnosis books define as mood disorder. Now that I understand the feelings associated with crappy would it be okay for me to check in with you about how crappy you have been feeling using that word?"

This process is essential when working with language related to sexuality and intimacy. Clients will often use slang because this is more comfortable for them or because it is the only terminology they know for their body or sexual behaviors. There are some specific goals related to language that we need to be mindful of in the process.

1.   Ask permission. Language is personal and we demonstrate respect and offer an opportunity for experiencing permission and consent with a client. "You used the word cunt. Do you prefer that word? Would it be alright if I use that word when we discuss topics around the body and sex?" It is important we always maintain a professional purpose in our work. We need to identify that sharing language is about comfort and choice.

2.   Provide education. We may be the first and only safe people to offer information. In order for our clients to receive help around their bodies and health they need a shared knowledge and language with medical providers. "You used the word cunt. Are you referring to the external part of genitals or the inside or both? Doctors might use the word labia, vulva, clitoris, penis, vagina to refer to genitals. Are you familiar with these terms? Do you prefer I use the term cunt when we talk about these topics?"

3.   Ensure comfort and reduce the power dynamic. When individuals feel comfortable in the topic of sexuality, they can be more open, and more work can get done. Insisting on specific, medically correct language can create more of the expert-receiver dynamic. Our goal is to empower the client regarding their sexuality and sexual experiences and that often begins owning their narrative.

It is important to note that sex educators and therapists have historically been taught to use medically correct language. I do believe that it is important to work from a space of education related to terminology, but I have found great benefit to negotiating language with clients rather than forcing something that can feel disconnected for a client.

Ensuring Client Does Not Have to Be Educator

It is impossible to be well-versed and informed on every topic. Being willing to talk about certain topics is not enough. We need to be familiar with the topics that are likely to be addressed, language that is used, and questions or comments that might be offensive.

Graduate studies provide a baseline knowledge for entering the field. It is our ethical responsibility to remain well-informed of changes to diagnosis, assessment, and intervention. It is our ethical responsibility to remain informed of health consequences and needs within specific communities we may serve. Having a strong network of professionals that can offer information and resources about a diversity of communities and practice approaches, is one of the best ways to ensure we remain educated and relevant in our field of practice.

When a topic is brought up that is new to us it is appropriate to acknowledge this with the client and ensure they know we will be doing our work to research the topic. Certainly, the internet is a place to start but not end. Journal and academic publications that offer recent research on topics are necessary. Expanding resources by investigating self-help books or instructional books on the topic and accessing referral sources and community resources related to certain topics is also important.

Professional Confidence

Remaining aware of the purpose and importance of discussing sexuality and intimacy is very important. It is not uncommon for clients to become overwhelmed or excited by discussing topics previously guarded. Sometimes clients will switch the focus to normalize or establish connection when there is a feeling of discomfort. Checking in may come in the form of attributing emotions to the clinician such as, "you probably think it is weird I like. . .?" Sometimes clients seek to decrease the discomfort by asking about the clinician's preferences or experiences such as, "you seem pretty open so you wouldn't describe yourself as just vanilla?" If we remain confident in our purpose, curious to understand the intention of the question or comment and consistent in establishing healthy boundaries, we can navigate these moments with success.

"A lot of folks find it fun and sometimes overwhelming to discuss these topics with someone else." A comment like this might open the door to helping the client identify what is coming up for them.

"Asking about my experiences and opinions is often a way to establish an understanding of what is 'normal' but the great thing about sexuality is there doesn't need to be a 'normal' it is open to what you want and need." A comment like this may reassure the client that there is no judgement from the clinician.

"Discussing your sexuality and experiences with another person can be really vulnerable. Remember you are in charge of what you share. Are you feeling safe to continue?" A question like this is a good reframe and opportunity to guide the discussion with consent.

"It makes a lot of sense that you would be curious about me and my experiences, but it is important to allow this space to be about you. It is one of the few relationships in life that you are encouraged to be selfish and enjoy connection and focus on your own experiences." A comment like this can help to establish boundaries.

Unlike discussing family history or symptoms of mental illness, topics of sexuality can feel unclear in their purpose. Our understanding of sexuality as a core domain of identity and functioning keeps the topic grounded. When the client becomes uncomfortable or unclear related to boundaries, it is imperative that we are capable of keeping the process safe and purposeful. We need to do this in a way that is not shaming but offers clarity.

Transference and Countertransference

Interpersonal practice work in all graduate education spends significant time defining transference and countertransference. We work to understand why it occurs and how to manage it in a healthy manner within the therapeutic relationship. Transference refers to a redirection of feelings about our desire for another person that belongs to an entirely different person. For instance, a feeling of energy and lightness toward a therapist because they have attributes that remind the client of their first best friend. The energy and lightness are feelings really about the best friend relationship but whatever the similarity, these feelings transfer to the therapist or therapist relationship. Because it is enjoyable, aspects of a past relationship would be referred to as positive transference. When a client experiences feelings of fearfulness and negativity toward the therapist because they speak in the same tone and gesture like the client's abusive father, this reminder is negative, thus negative transference (Teyber & Teyber, 2017).

Another type of transference is erotic transference. Erotic transference is positive transference accompanied by sexual fantasies that the client understands to be unrealistic. The fantasies do not interfere with the motivation for therapeutic purpose or goals. This may be directly discussed by the client with the therapist. The therapist may notice behavior that might be considered flirtatious and see this as an opportunity to revisit purpose of the work and importance of the therapeutic relationship and boundaries that keep the relationship unique, safe, and important. Erotic transference is fairly common and makes sense because of the vulnerability and emotional intimacy of the therapeutic relationship (Ladson & Welton, 2007). Exploring sexuality and intimacy in detail may heighten the possibility of erotic transference. It can feel new and different to speak with such openness with someone. It is not a problem in and of itself, as long as the therapist is capable of addressing the transference, setting boundaries, and never creating shame for the client. Key to erotic transference is the understanding held by the client that the fantasies are unrealistic (Stefana, 2017).

A client I had seen for several months started a session having a hard time with eye contact and seeming especially restless. I asked if they were doing alright, noting these differences in behavior. The client shared, "I feel really weird and uncomfortable telling you this but . . . I keep having dreams we are having sex. Sometimes, I actually enjoy them and I really feel this is messed up."

I felt a bit nervous because I really wanted to handle this effectively. I had studied erotic transference and discussed it with supervisors, so I felt confident addressing the issue. I shared with the client my appreciation for their honesty. I shared my sincere belief that they weren't doing something weird or wrong. I shared my understanding that the therapeutic relationship is a unique relationship that allows openness and unconditional positive regard, is devoted completely to the needs of the client and is based in protective boundaries that ensure the stability of the relationship and the needs of the client as the only priority. I asked the client if there was anything that felt uncomfortable or confusing about our interaction.

The client released a big sigh and expressed relief that they had told me and that I wasn't uncomfortable. They reflected that talking about all the difficult emotions and having me listen and care was different for them and that it did bring up a lot of feelings. We agreed to continue checking in often to make sure the therapy space and relationship felt predictable and safe.

Very different from this example is the case of Eroticized Transference. This is defined by intense, vivid, irrational, and erotic preoccupation with the therapist. Even with effort from the therapist, the client cannot develop appropriate insights and is motivated to have closeness with the therapist rather than motivation for therapeutic goals. It is likely that this type of transference can only be defined after the therapist has made an effort to clarify roles and boundaries. However, the behavior of the client is generally forward, if not demanding from the start. This may cause discomfort and red flags for the therapist. It is most often the case that the therapist's efforts cannot create change with eroticized transference, and it is best to refer the client to another provider.

A client I worked with in residential placement often suggested that I must find him attractive. He shared sexual fantasies about me and refused redirection or clarification that this was not realistic. He interpreted basic social interactions as simple as a smile or expression of concern as "a secret message." Efforts to clarify boundaries were increasingly met with anger and demands. The intensity, irrationality, and lack of change, despite efforts for boundary setting and clarification, are hallmarks of eroticized transference. It was necessary for him to move out of the residential treatment group I directed. I met with him a final time, with another treatment staff present, and clarified the reason we couldn't work together, the importance of him continuing to receive help that would allow him to focus on his own important therapy goals without distraction. Despite the difficulty of the interactions, I had with this client I did my best not to create shame in the ending of the therapeutic relationship.

As clinicians we hold enormous responsibility for maintaining our role and boundaries with clients to ensure clarity of the work and safety of the relationship. Many of our clients have been mistreated, used, manipulated in relationships and they very much need the safety of therapy to heal. It is quite common for therapists to experience countertransference. Best practices are to have consistent self-care in the work and to notice signs of countertransference and seek change or support.

Personal Reflection

The following list represents tasks and rituals that are important behaviors for self-care. Check off the items you have done in the last week. Note how many times in the week you have participated in the behavior. If you check off less than five items, make a note of what is hindering you in your life from these behaviors. Do you have a way of justifying this self-neglect? If so, how can you challenge this justification?

Finishing work in the office/not taking work home

Sleeping seven to eight hours a night

Leaving work on time

Participating in a hobby

Journaling

Communicating with friends unrelated to the helping profession

Communicating with supervisor

Communicating with colleagues

Exercise

Meditation

Creation (form of expressive art)

Add your own if it is not listed:

How many times a week?

What is hindering you from self-care?

How do you justify self-neglect?

How can you challenge the justification?

Warning Signs That Therapists Are Experiencing/Acting on Countertransference

Modifying appearance because you are seeing a client

Meeting with client at the end of the day or before a lunch break so you can go over time

Offering additional access that is not provided for most clients

Sharing about self beyond useful disclosure

Thinking about client outside of sessions

It is important to be aware of our emotions, our countertransference, so we can respond in helpful ways. It is often a sign that there is not enough support or emotional stimulation in life outside of work, so the therapist is trying to meet personal needs through work. Increasing connection with friends, family, partner, communicating about countertransference with supervisor and increasing self-care are always ways to stay within boundaries and role.

Clarity of our values and mission in our work as well as our role with clients will help us to navigate many difficult scenarios that can come up in the course of work. Interpersonal Practice work is multifaceted and requires an intense self-awareness. Knowing and caring for ourselves is a critical part of the work that often does not receive the attention it requires during graduate studies. Challenge that trend!

Questions for Reflection and Discussion

Briefly evaluate your own self-care. Are there aspects that are lacking? Can you commit to any improvements?

When you consider professional confidence and discussing sexuality and intimacy with clients, what ages, identities or populations feel most difficult to raise the topic with? Why?

Collaborative Assessment Strategies

5

Introduction

The biopsychosocial assessment is a common tool used by many mental health practitioners. Some agencies may utilize standard intake forms, as well as standardized tools for assessment related to specific diagnosis. The collaborative relationship of Interpersonal Practice work, and the understanding of the person in society as a key element of our clinical framework, results in most clinical social workers utilizing a narrative approach to gather information. To review, the domains of functioning explored in a biopsychosocial assessment include:

Presenting Problem

- Signs and symptoms resulting in impairment
- Current examples of symptoms in multiple domains of functioning: social, occupational, affective, cognitive, physical
- History of presenting problem, events, precipitating factors or incidents leading to need for services
- Frequency/duration/severity/cycling of symptoms
- Time when symptoms worsened

Family Mental Health History

- Diagnosed mental illness
- Symptoms of mental illness in family (diagnosed and undiagnosed)

DOI: 10.4324/9781003166382-6

- Substance use disorder
- Generational trauma (history of traumatic events)

Current Family/Significant Relationship

- Strengths/supports
- Stressors/problems
- Recent changes
- Changes desired

Childhood/Adolescent History

- Developmental milestones
- Past behavioral concerns
- Environment
- Abuse
- School
- Social
- Mental health

Cultural/Ethnic

- Strengths/supports
- Stressors/problems
- Beliefs/practices

Spiritual/Religious

- Strengths/supports
- Stressors/problems
- Beliefs/practices
- Recent changes
- Changes desired

Legal

- History
- Status/impact/stressors

Education

- Strengths
- Weaknesses

- Socio-relational/peer relationships
- Learning difficulties

Employment/Vocational

- Strengths/supports
- Stressors/problems

Leisure/Recreational

- Strengths
- Recent changes
- Changes desired

Physical Health

- Summary of health
- Physical factors affecting mental condition
- Experience interacting with medical health profession

Chemical Use History

- Summary of use
- Type of substances
- Frequency of use
- Client's perception of problem

Counseling Prior to Treatment

- Summary of prior treatment
- Benefits
- Setbacks

It is noticeable that sexuality and intimacy is missing from the standard biopsychosocial. In the last decade, sexuality is sometimes included as a domain with the assessment and often includes:

Sexuality

- Orientation
- Prior experiences
- Abuse/trauma
- Current experience

Even when we find sexuality included as a domain, it is often limited in the information we assess and how we understand the relationship of sexuality to the other domains of functioning. When I gather information about medical health, and a person shares that they have diabetes, I am trained to consider how relational stressors impact physical wellness as well as adherence to diabetes treatment. It seems very reasonable to assume that diabetes can influence the functioning of the body and the ability to engage in sexual experiences. What is missing is our comfort in discussing this and forming these connections related to overall health and functioning during our assessment process.

A sexual health assessment covers all domains of a person's sexuality, including gender, orientation, sexual experiences, and current sexual health and intimacy status.

Presenting Problem/Concern

    Description of the problem

    Onset of the problem

    Understanding of why the problem exists

    Past efforts to address problem

Social Information

    Family of origin

    Attachment relationship with attachment figures in childhood

    Influential peer relationships during childhood and adolescence

    Peer relations/history of mistreatment or bullying

    Resiliency and coping mechanisms

    Influential life experiences

    Social interests past and current

    Present home and family dynamics

    Capacity to experience pleasure in life

Health Data

    Current experiences of pain and wellness

    History of illness

    Family history of illness

    Availability of resources to care for health

Use of nutrition, movement

Sleep hygiene

Current medications-access and use

Use of substances

Thought and mood: ruminations, anxiety, depression, obsessions/compulsions, panic

Employment History

Current experience in workplace

Future goals

Disappointments

Financial Concerns

Ability to care for basic needs

Ability to plan for future needs

Affordability of pleasure opportunities (gifts, vacations, etc.)

Communication of finances in relationship/household

Level of stress related to financial decisions/debt

Gender/orientation/relational history

Were there open or unacknowledged sexual minorities, or gender minority people in your family, community, school?

What was your family's attitude toward sexual or gender minorities?

What effect do you think your family has had on your own sexuality and sexual relationships?

Are there rituals related to gender and sexuality specific to your religion or culture that you participated in while growing up

Sexual History

Earliest remembered sexual experiences and general attitude about them

How sex was learned about

How sex was discussed by adults

How sex was discussed with peers

Developmental changes and emotional responses to changes

Influential experiences during childhood, adolescence, and adulthood related (trauma experiences may be presented without acknowledgement of impact)

Age of awareness of sexual orientation and response of loved ones/peers

Any shame or negative reaction related to sexual orientation, gender expression or sexual habits/practices during development

Sexual mistreatment/negative sexual experiences

Experiences of masturbation

Experiences of orgasm and ejaculation

Difficulty with menses/pregnancy/births/terminations of pregnancies/infertility

How have children affected sense of sexual self and sex life

General current attitude about sex and its importance in life

Self-concept as a sexual person

Decisions about safer sex and birth control

Current status of sexuality and intimacy

Are there difficulties related to lack of interest, premature ejaculation, getting/keeping an erection, foreplay, reaching orgasm, pain?

Do you feel affirmed in your gender and orientation within your relationship during sexual activity?

Decisions and communication about monogamy/non-monogamy

Motivation to make changes

How frequent is intimacy experienced?

How is intimacy negotiated

Is penetrative sex occurring, is it important, is it enjoyable

Are there sexual experiences that are wanted/preferred that are not currently happening?

Range of sexual behaviors and comfort level

Are there aspects of sexual identity they have not been able to incorporate into current relationship or practices?

(Foley et al., 2012; Cavanaugh, 2019)

This assessment format may look like an overwhelming amount of information. It is common that topics overlap and result in a conversational experience of assessment. Ideally, the assessment process offers new insight and reflection for the client, rather than simply data gathering. This is especially true when clients are invited to discuss relationships and development and incorporate their sexual identity. A successful assessment should deliver some "aha moments" that illustrate patterns/themes or "the thread" that connects past to present.

The Thread

Assessment information is gathered in an effort to build rapport and develop a case conceptualization. As we use questions to prompt discussion of social, relational history we listen closely to identify patterns and themes that weave within domains of functioning. In teaching I refer to this as *the thread*. If we imagine a weaving or fabric knitted together, we can see that, at first glance, it is viewed as a whole piece. By looking closely, we can identify individual threads woven throughout the piece. That thread serves to join, to hold together, and of course sometimes becomes hidden or tangled within the fabric. When we look closely and find *the thread*, we can understand the entire person more and we can sometimes help to untangle, reweave.

The following example demonstrates this process of case conceptualization or understanding *the thread* of patterns and themes.

Case Study: Janice

Janice enters the assessment identifying presenting problems with low motivation, lack of pleasure, decreased energy, and poor communication with husband and family of origin. She doesn't feel listened to or understood in her relationship with her husband, mother or father. She notes that she has patterns of attempted communication that lead to volatility and then gives up and retreats into decreased communication and a bit of isolation.

She is the oldest of five siblings and her mother parented them mostly alone throughout the client's childhood. Her mother had a series of relationships with men that fell short of support or success. This left the client with sadness for her mother and frustration with her mother. Many of her friends have been lifelong friends that experienced similar events in development including parental divorce, unfulfilling dating relationships in teenage years and financial struggles throughout their lives. Janice experiences support through these relationships but the struggles she has faced are normalized within her peer support group and not often recognized as something that could be better or different.

She expresses that daily life feels without pleasure. She doesn't feel appreciation for the things she does, and things feel like they lack meaning and purpose. Her husband doesn't often talk to her about the things that are meaningful to her. He works many hours and leaves most of the household and child rearing responsibilities to her. In comparison to her friends and her mother, she feels she should be grateful for the consistency and financial security offered by her husband.

She was recently diagnosed with fibromyalgia as well as having a history of irritable bowel syndrome. The lack of energy and motivation has definitely negatively impacted self-care related to nutrition and exercise.

She notes that an unexpected pregnancy caused her to drop out of college and get married. Even though she truly loves being a mother she is sad about not being able to complete her college experience and develop her own career path. Her husband holds a well-paying position and they do not have current debt or financial difficulties.

She notes that she has had a series of unfulfilling romantic relationships. She had little support or education related to sex, boys, and dating. The question about shame opens floodgates of tears and Janice shares a story of sexual assault that occurred when she was 14 years of age. She has told only her friends who offered support by sharing similar experiences. Anxiety, low mood, and low self-worth followed this traumatic event. She has always managed sexual experiences by drinking "a bit too much" to get through it. She has had a series of unwanted sexual experiences and unfulfilling experiences throughout adolescent and young adult years. The lack of support or ability to receive comfort from her mother causes deep sadness and resentment. It makes her feel distant from her husband that he doesn't know any of her history. She doesn't describe her current sexual experiences as nonconsensual but she lacks self-awareness of her own desire and does not communicate at all regarding her needs or wants. Sex once a week is a way to "get through" and give her husband what she thinks he wants. She isn't sure how much it impacts her mood but notes there is a constant tension in her body.

Janice notes that she feels disconnected from her most important relationships as well as disconnected from her own body. She notes that she has always wanted to feel uninhibited and to experience pleasure. This has always felt like something out of her reach that only happens for other women. She notes that after the sexual assault in early adolescence, she experienced years of unhealthy relationships. She had little emotional or sexual safety or pleasure. She connects drinking too much alcohol as a way to numb and create a "pretend normal." When she met her husband, he seemed so "normal" that she "played the part" as a wife that would suit him because she didn't want to seem "damaged."

The thread:

> **Lack of safety**: The sexual assault early in adolescence resulted in a series of relationships that caused emotional and sexual harm. In her present life, she often feels triggered by sexual experiences with her husband but ignores and disconnects to "get through."

> **Lack of support**: Her mother did not support her with sexual education or emotional closeness that would have allowed her to feel safe to disclose her assaults. Her sadness and physical pain (fibromyalgia) were often minimized or ignored by her father, mother, and husband.

> **Numb/Disconnect**: The lack of support and resources to address her trauma caused her to disconnect from her body and push away the trauma. Alcohol and dissociation became a way to cope.

> **"Ah ha" moment**: The sexual pain she experienced has been shame-filled and resulted in a disconnection from her own body. The disempowerment and lack of communication related to her sexual feelings made her feel unseen by her family, especially husband. She carried a deep resentment in the relationship and was reminded of her unhealed trauma on a regular basis when she forced herself to have sex with her husband. Much of the tension she held in her body had manifested in physical symptoms presenting as fibromyalgia.

We will return to Janice's story in Chapter 11 in discussion of treatment interventions.

When considering assessment, a great rule of thumb is that the best assessments also serve as interventions to some degree. The long assessment paperwork that requires clients to checklist experiences that have occurred and dates/ages of these experiences rarely develops insights and are often triggering.

Sexual Health Timeline

The sexual health timeline can be used as a less formal approach to assessment. A series of questions that follow development benchmarks and common experiences that occur in the lifespan can offer a reflective experience of personal assessment that is then processed in the therapy context.

Introducing the sexual health timeline might include the idea of understanding influential events that occurred related to the development of the client's sexuality. The client can be prompted to share experiences they remember, were told about or sometimes reflect on neglect of experience/information or what needed to happen that didn't happen.

Early Childhood

What gender were you assigned at birth? (male/female/intersex)

Were there any concerns about your gender/genitals when you were born?

First awareness of gender and your gender. Did this match what you were assigned at birth?

First awareness of genitals

First awareness that different people had different types of genitals

Mid Childhood

First sexual sensation

First sex play with same-age peers

Initial discussions with parents or other adults about sex

Initial discussion with other children about sex

First time you touched yourself in a pleasurable way/masturbated

Sex education in school

Curiosity about sexual behavior

Seeing sexual behavior on-line, on television, in print

Were you ever mistreated or bullied based on gender or orientation in childhood?

Adolescence – Young Adulthood

First menstruation

First memory of erection

How did others react to your body changing? How did you feel about the reactions?

Learning sexual slang

First noticing changes in secondary sex characteristics

Did you try to hide these changes or feel shame about them?

Did your gender presentation and behavior match expectations peers/ family have for you?

First daydreams or fantasies that were sexual

Doing something that is considered "bad" sexually

What feelings did you have about attractions or other indicators of sexual orientation?

Did you experience conflict between your sexual behavior and the lessons of religion or cultural identity?

Did you have an experience of 'coming out' or sharing any part of your sexual orientation or gender identity?

First time being touched in a sexual way (negative or positive experience)

First time touching another in a sexual way (negative or positive experience)

Feeling of attraction to another person

First kiss

First time touching another's body

First time viewing pornography

First time being touched on anus, chest, genitals digitally or orally

First time touching another's anus, chest, genitals digitally or orally

First penetrative sexual experience

First time using substances while being sexual

Adulthood

Making decisions related to safer sex (contraception, PREP, etc.)

Contracting an STI

First gynecological exam

Difficulty with sexual "performance" (erection, lubrication, etc.)

Pay or type of exchange for sexual behavior

Pregnancy

Abortion

Exploration of BDSM

Exploration of Kink

Opening up relationship

Beginning polyamorous relationships

Using sex toys solo or with partner

Describing specific sexual needs to a partner

Sex after childbirth

Sex during perimenopause

Additional topics included in transgender assessment:

Realized you didn't fit into the boy/girl categories you were "supposed" to?

Were you scolded or punished for not behaving like your gender assigned at birth?

The first time you felt shame or embarrassment of expressing yourself in a way that did not align with your gender assigned at birth?

What do you remember about initial signs of puberty (breast development, nocturnal emission, hair growth, voice change)?

How did family or friends react to initial signs of puberty?

Who did you first talk to about your gender identity? How did they react?

What reactions did you experience from school, community, family, peers?

Did you experience threats or violence?

Did you often feel unsafe?

What did you rely on to cope?

(Foley, Kope, Sugrue, 2012)

You may not need to complete a sexuality timeline and a sexual health assessment. Consider your client as well as the timing of your setting. The timeline may be a reflective activity that your client can work on outside of session and bring to session to discuss. Be cautious of how overwhelming these questions may be and remember to frame the work. Framing the timeline would include (1) purpose: to reflect and build insight regarding how past experiences influence your current sexual attitude (2) pacing: we don't often think about these memories with great intention so it can be overwhelming and important to take a break (how will you take a break?) (3) caution: you may uncover information that you have not ever processed and this may be very difficult. A client that shows interest and willingness toward reflection related to their sexuality may be a good candidate to work independently on the sexuality timeline. A client that is guarded, has identified sexual trauma or feels uncomfortable with the initial questions related to sexuality may be better served by exploring the broader questions of the sexual health assessment in the session.

As mentioned earlier, the best assessment tool can gather data and also serve as an intervention. After a client has completed a sexuality timeline some considerations are useful. Begin by highlighting experiences that felt negative or positive. This often may be related to how others reacted versus the experience itself. Discussing in more detail some of these experiences can help clients to reflect on resiliency and it can also allow for grieving. Listen for grief of what did occur and negative or harmful experiences. Also listen for the grief of what did not occur that was needed or wanted. Reflecting on future expectations or the idea of the sexual self you are becoming may instill hope and allow the client to incorporate new insights into elements of treatment planning.

Body Reflection

There are many presenting problems that require a greater assessment and insight into the client's relationship to their body. Eating disorders, self-harm, history of emotional, physical or sexual abuse, body dysmorphia, gender dysphoria to name just a few presenting issues that are rather directly connected to the body and the person's relationship to their body.

When we ask clients to engage in a somatic assessment or body reflection, we generally want to introduce the concept. We can do this by referencing:

- the beliefs we hold about our bodies often influence how we negotiate being treated or communicating about our physical or sexual needs
- helping to be aware of and improve our messaging about our bodies can increase pleasure, relaxation, and decrease pain
- insight about our bodies can help us increase skills related to mindfulness and visualization that are evidence-based, to aid in pain management, recovery, concentration, management of anxiety and many more presenting conditions

Be cautious introducing body assessments because avoidance can be a common coping mechanism. Notice your client's reaction to the proposal of body-based assessment and respond gradually with opportunities for processing emotions if avoidance or expression of being overwhelmed is noted.

Mindfulness: Body Scan

A good place to start in body-centered work is completing a guided meditation with your client. For individuals that have had trauma occur to their body, mindfulness centered on the body, can be overwhelming. It can be helpful to begin with a generalized mindfulness on a part of the body. Peter Levine, creator of Somatic Experiencing, a body-informed psychotherapy practice guides clients in this way:

> Place a hand on your forehead and the other hand over your heart. Close your eyes if comfortable and focus on the sensations in the area of your body between your two hands. Bring awareness into this area of your body and notice temperature, sensations of tension, tingling, ease . . . (allow 2 minutes). Move your hand from your forehead to your gut, leaving the other hand over your heart. Again, focus on the sensations in the area of your body between your two hands. Bring awareness into this area of your body and notice temperature, sensations of tension, tingling, ease. . . (allow 2 minutes).
>
> (Levine, 1999)

This is a great way to give a client brief exposure to this type of activity. It allows them to practice and hopefully feel safe in the activity. You may then incorporate a more detailed guided visualization in the form of a body scan. A body scan can last from three minutes to 15–20 minutes. The level of detail naming each part of the body, and allowing time for the client to visualize it, can influence how much time is dedicated. For example, "bring awareness to your forehead, then cheeks, then mouth" or "bring awareness to your head."

Body Map

Using expressive therapy, you can ask a client to draw a picture of parts of their body they like or dislike. The client can also name and share descriptive words of certain body parts. This allows clients to discuss the areas that feel safe to discuss.

A client might also draw a life-size outline of their body and then have them trace the actual body outline on that same paper. There is generally a discrepancy in the size and shape of body parts or overall size that can be reflect on.

Introducing the mirror exercise is advised for most individuals. You can ask someone to begin for five minutes timed in front of a mirror looking at their face. Encourage them to write down words they noticed or sensations in their body. For some, specific memories may come about.

Gradually expand exposure gauging client's reaction. For many experiences of trauma and difficult emotions may surface. Ways to approach in steps include:

> Beginning with head, expand to top arms and chest, etc.
>
> Beginning with clothes on and gradually removing clothes

This activity will be discussed in more detail in Chapter 11 of this book.

DOUPE

An assessment algorithm designed by AASECT Sex Therapist Sallie Foley gathers information about resiliency and subjective experience and to highlight pleasure over performance. The assessment algorithm known as DOUPE approaches questions in this framework:

(D) Description of the problem

(O) Onset of the problem

(U) Client understanding of why the problem exists

(P) Past experiences addressing the problem

(E) Expectations for treatment

A lead-in request to the series of questions we are labeling DOUPE: "tell me about a recent sexual experience." As the individual describes the experience, we may begin to use the DOUPE questions to tweak our understanding of the problem. The following case example captures the DOUPE assessment:

> The DOUPE questions can be used as a stand-alone in an informal assessment experience or within the sexual health assessment to gather important information related to the presenting problem. It is common to use these questions during on-going clinical conversations with

clients. It is important to note that assessment is a continual experience, as the therapeutic relationship develops and as an individual gains trust and insight more information is shared that may require investigation.

(Foley, 2015)

Here is a case example utilizing the DOUPE model of assessment:

Case Study: Hazel

When working with Hazel, a 65-year-old, cisgender, white woman in a monogamous relationship for 42 years with same man, additional information was presented organically, and we used the DOUPE assessment to gather information.

When talking about a family visit Hazel commented that it was surprising how open her granddaughters and nieces were about their body and sex. She mentioned that they talked about orgasms and reflected some sadness that she would never know what that would be like. I clarified with Hazel and asked her if intimacy with herself or with her partner was enjoyable.

Hazel shared that they didn't have sex anymore because "I guess it gets painful" around 40. I asked her if she would feel comfortable sharing what intimacy was like before they stopped. Hazel said that her husband, Stan, would always join her in bed and tap her shoulder. "This was a sign that he wanted to have sex," she explained. She would roll over toward him and he would kiss her on the mouth a bit. Earlier in the relationship he had wanted to do "things down there" but she didn't feel that was comfortable. So, after kissing they would try for penetration.

I asked, "when it started hurting, can you DESCRIBE the pain?" Hazel shared that it pinched a lot when it started to go in and then hurt tremendously when it was all the way in. I clarified, "the pain didn't start until sometime in your 40s?" Hazel shared that the onset was around 44 years of age and she had started to notice "the change" in reference to perimenopause. Before the pain, there wasn't a lot of pleasure but no pain. At this point we have the description of pain and the *onset* of pain. We could choose to learn more about the lack of orgasm or pleasure but, according to Hazel, she chose to stop intimacy and has some regrets about what didn't occur, and the reason she stopped is related to pain.

I continue to assess by asking, "Why do you think the pain started?" Based on my understanding of Hazel and the description of her biological experience

I can certainly develop my own hypothesis, but it is very important to gather the *understanding* of the presenting problem from the client's perspective. Hazel responds, "I think I just got all dried up from getting older." This allows me to find out if there is anything she did to address the problem based on what she understood was wrong. Hazel shares that she tried putting some water on her finger and inserting the water inside her vagina, but this didn't make any improvements. Her husband suggested they could "warm up" a little but again this felt uncomfortable to Hazel, so she didn't pursue that idea. Finding out what has been tried to address the problem is referred to as the past experience.

Finally, I ask Hazel if the pain could be addressed, would she still want intimacy in her life with herself or her husband. She laughed at the possibility of addressing the pain and then said, "why of course, we miss that. It was the only time I really felt close and loved." As I assess the expectations, I might want to find out more specifically what type of intimacy is expected. For Hazel I surmised that her understanding of options was limited and I might want to dedicate some psychoeducation to this issue as a treatment approach.

My interaction with Hazel took place in the context of a 60-minute therapy session and certainly deepened my understanding of her life and her relationship. Hazel was a self-sacrificer and often felt unloved, resentful, and spread thin from all the giving. The context of our work was about having and communicating expectations as well as setting boundaries. It is clear how the experience of intimacy reflects these larger life themes of self-sacrifice, lack of communication of needs. I also felt hopeful that helping Hazel explore this element of herself may be empowering and helping her return to sexual intimacy with her husband might help her feel more connected and loved.

The DOUPE assessment is easy to remember and offers a thorough assessment of any presenting problem, especially sexual health and intimacy difficulties. It is informal and generally allows clients to be thoughtful about life before the problem (onset question), which can stimulate ideas about underlying causes in their life. Using Hazel as an example, there was some awareness that her body changes influenced the pain experience, even though she did not have information about the body's natural lubrication or store-bought lubrication.

The assessment strategies offered in this chapter are all interactive in processing opportunities for collaboration, reflection, and the growth of insight. They allow us to connect information about attachment experiences, both in childhood and peer/partnered relationships. They include information about biological and medical experiences, trauma, and grief. As the field of social work and mental health develops into a more integrated field with a stronger somatic focus, it is important to be prepared to use assessment centered in the body. While some of the examples offered in this chapter may feel different for clients, I encourage you to embrace the opportunity and lead with confidence. Chapter 11 will connect these assessment approaches with common interventions.

Questions for Reflection and Discussion

Using the concept of the thread, what are some patterns/themes that you notice in clients you are working with in your internship? Have you been able to identify this with your clients? Is there a connection to their sexual self?

How are these collaborative assessment strategies different from the current assessment strategies you are learning about in other classes or using at your internship? What are benefits/drawbacks?

Trauma and Sexual Difficulties

6

Introduction

The last two decades of neuroscience and integrated care have dramatically changed clinicians' understanding of stressors, trauma, the body and regulation. The information has shaped approaches to trauma assessment and healing. We have learned that there is the trauma we *know*, the trauma we *hold* and sometimes it is both. References to holding trauma relates to the expression of trauma on the body system and functioning.

In sex therapy, we understand a direct correlation to trauma and experiences of sexuality and intimacy. In social work services, clinicians often struggle with incorporating the current experience into the trauma healing process. This is crucial because the individual must be able to modify their trauma narrative and understand how it has changed them as a person, including as a sexual person. Some of these changes may be related to Post Traumatic Resilience and relate to the change of self. For others, this may relate to Post Traumatic Growth and they may feel empowered by their trauma experience to embody a new way of knowing and expressing their sexual self. In the course of that healing journey, we need to parallel trauma processing with tools to understand their current sexuality and relational sexual experiences.

Stages of healing as defined by psychiatrist and author Judith Herman include establishment of safety, remembrance, and mourning, and reconnection. Herman's research identified disempowerment and disconnection from others, as core experiences of trauma. Connection and relationship, both to the clinician and expanding to create healthy connections in community, are

DOI: 10.4324/9781003166382-7

key to healing. Restoration of connection is where the recreation and healing of trust, autonomy, initiative, competence, identity, and intimacy exist. Trauma healing, identified by Herman and shared by most trauma-informed specialists, honors the importance of power and control as central to the *process* of healing. Decision making, boundary setting, pacing, and permission-giving are routine in the process of interaction with the client and reinforce the empowerment and control of the individual to have control over the content and experience of healing (Herman, 1995).

Using the summary chart in Table 6.1, we can think about what issues of sexuality and intimacy may surface during each stage of healing. There are different topics to focus on in each stage. Remembering, of course, healing stages are not always "one and done," and often reality causes individuals to return to earlier stages.

What to listen for:

Hypo/hypersexual behavior are both associated with trauma.

Attachment Theory has long influenced interpersonal practice work. From Attachment Theory we know that the ways people initially recognized (or did not) and responded to (effectively or ineffectively) our basic needs for nurture, care, and connection influences our ability to recognize and respond to our own needs. Attachment experiences that require our avoidance of needs sometimes results in being in a hypo-regulated space. In Polyvagal Theory, a neurophysiological theory of regulation, it is referred to as a dorsal state. Attachment experiences that are painful and label our needs as a problem or responds to them in unpredictable ways result in specific ways of coping. It may result in learning to calm these needs through means that are not connection but rather through excess behaviors or being in a hyper-regulated state, or Sympathetic State, as it is referred to in Polyvagal Theory (Dana, 2020).

It is important to note that most clients will not have a great deal of insight into why their sexual behaviors are dysregulated but may be able to describe a sense of being "shut down" (hypo/dorsal state) or operating "like a motor" (hyper/sympathetic state) instead of feeling directed by the flow of sensation and emotions. Many clients have described that "there is a hard switch rather than a dial" to manage sexual feelings/needs/sensations.

A dislike or disconnection of one's body is also common. The relationship to one's body, how it is treated, fixated on, neglected or ignored can often alert us to trauma that is unspoken in the assessment process. It can also help us connect a known trauma to how the system is managing, experiencing, and holding the trauma. Examples of dislike, or disconnection of one's body, might be depriving the body of food, movement, hygiene, sleep, medication.

Table 6.1 Aligning Trauma Treatment with Sexuality and Intimacy Treatment

	Establishment of Safety	**Remembrance and Mourning**	**Reconnection**
Trauma Tx Goals	Gathering history and understanding current triggers. Establishing safety in one's self through boundaries, regulation, somatic, and mindfulness experiences.	Naming traumatic experiences. Connecting current beliefs, thoughts, emotions, behaviors to traumatic experiences. Grieving what did not occur in the space that trauma did occur.	Reconnecting to experiences and people. Sometimes this may include sharing your experience with others or connecting with others that are also healing.
Sexuality/ Intimacy Issues	Identifying current beliefs and behaviors that may be reinforcing sexual fear, avoidance, powerlessness. Establishing concepts related to consent. Regulating hypo/hyper sex expression that may be tied to trauma versus pleasure. Practice listening to messages about emotional and physical comfort, safety, pleasure.	Identifying ways that sexual trauma has influenced beliefs about body and pleasure. Identifying themes of safety and trust in intimacy with current or new partners. Identifying ways, the body and mind may re-experience lack of safety, fear, pain in current experiences.	Reconnecting to self, one's body or to others in new ways. Experiencing empowerment and/or pleasure.

This table shows the trauma treatment goals and sexuality issues that correlate with each of the three phases of Judith Herman's stages of healing.

It could also include self-harm or lack of safety in situations, decision-making that puts a person at risk (Fontanesi et al., 2021).

In our initial assessment process, it is important to understand daily functioning. It assists us in the diagnosis process. Individuals have often normalized symptoms of trauma, therefore broad questions such as, "do you feel well on a daily basis?" or "do you sleep well?" are not particularly beneficial. Here is a list of questions I ask to dig in a bit deeper to functioning and uncover symptoms related to diagnosis. It often serves to illustrate a disconnect from one's body that is telling of trauma experience.

SS. 1. Tell me about a typical day of your life from start to finish. (I'm listening for all the "boring" details such as time they wake up, how they wake up, do they eat alone or with others, etc.)

Things to listen for: isolation, avoidance behaviors, lack of routine, too much/ too little or dysregulation.

2. How does your body feel when you start your day?

Things to listen for: lack awareness or disconnection from sensations, chronic discomfort without diagnosis or treatment.

3. How does your body feel as you are sitting here now?

What parts feel good and where is their discomfort, pain, ache, tension?

Things to listen for: lack of awareness, defensiveness or discomfort being in touch with the body. Sometimes a very brief body scan can be helpful but requires consent and may be overwhelming for many clients.

4. Do you have opportunities to care for your body? This might include a warm shower, putting on lotion, a massage, yoga, etc.

Things to listen for: lack of pleasure attending to needs of the body, lack of insight regarding basic needs of body such as hygiene.

5. What is sleep like for you?

Do you feel tired throughout your day?

Do you feel rested when you wake up?

Do you fall asleep easily or find it difficult?

How long does it take to fall asleep?

Do you wake often throughout your sleep?

Things to listen for: consistent fatigue, restlessness, avoidance of sleep, excess sleep for comfort and avoidance.

6. Do you have resources and opportunities to nourish yourself throughout your day?

Do you enjoy eating?

Do you have time to eat?

Do you share meals or eat alone?

Things to listen for: neglect, deprivation, excess, lack of awareness of hunger/ fullness.

7. Do you take medications?

Do you have difficulty taking medications?

Are there often occasions when you skip medications and for what reason?

Things to listen for: uncertainty or discomfort with medication due to stigma of diagnosis, feeling undeserving of feeling better.

8. Do you receive / give touch often?

What is that like for you?

Do you enjoy this?

Is it too much or not enough?

Things to listen for: avoidance, lack of ownership of one's body, lack of consent, doing out of expectations or feeling programmed without interest or desire.

It is important to recognize that when the basic relationship with our own body is interrupted by traumatic experiences, we do not consciously choose behaviors that may be neglectful or harmful. These behaviors are an expression of the trauma on the body (Driscoll & Flanagan, 2016). Opening up this conversation in assessment often helps the client reflect concern or difficulty. It can most often create curiosity for why this is occurring. The curiosity is the piece we lean into in the clinical space to understand "the thread" between what is happening here / now. We also seek to understand how it came to be or how it relates to past events. This information leads to, most importantly, how to heal it.

Moving from curiosity to insight / from current to past

> "Noticing," being curious or observing, are common interpersonal skills woven into most therapeutic modalities. These are so important for empowering a client to look more deeply into something that they may feel is overwhelming or shame-based. It is empowering because the mental health professional is not claiming expertise, rather aligning beside the client in being curious about. . . or noticing that.

When do you use noticing?

• To bring attention to something that feels important: "I notice that eating a full meal doesn't happen on days you spend with your mother and father." Or "I'm noticing you frowning as you discuss giving your partner a hug when you get home."

• To increase insight or reflection: This is especially useful if you have a hypothesis and would like to explore it. "I notice you have kept to yourself a lot since your friend was assaulted."

When do you use exploration or "being curious?"

• To request a client, pay attention to a certain emotion or sensation. "I'm curious about how skipping dinner feels in your stomach?" Or "You said you don't feel anything during the body scan. Can we be curious about what purpose, feeling nothing, might have for your body?"

As insight increases through "noticing" and exploration or "being curious about" we can try to build a timeline of when these symptoms, patterns or relationship with the body started. At this point we have developed a bit of insight into the experience or meaning of the behavior and are tracking *the thread* to the past. Helpful questions to begin a timeline include:

- Do you remember a time when it was ever different? (You can insert the specific symptom or behavior such as skipping meals, isolating.)
- What do you remember about the timeframe within which this behavior started?

I often place a line in the middle of a blank piece of paper and place the behavior/symptom discussed toward the right side and label this "now" or "current." Any information a client can provide about the behavior being different in the past I would then mark on the timeline. Here on Figure 6.1, is a brief example of a client timeline.

A timeline reads left to right the events of an individual's life: (10) ate lots of candy alone while my dad was drinking, (15) parents divorced, binging started, (18–20) abusive relationship (two years) started cutting, (now) lack of self-care and lots of sex when drunk.

The events that may have been occurring before a behavior changed may point to a traumatic event that has been overlooked. A client may not mention it because they didn't find it relevant or thought they had already addressed it. The protocol for Eye Movement Desensitization Reprocessing (EMDR) developed by Francine Shapiro considers three clinical themes related to pervasive distortions and traumatic memory. These themes are: Responsibility/Defectiveness ("I am the cause of the

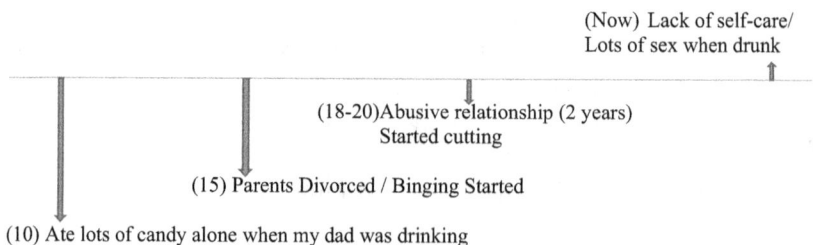

(Now) Lack of self-care/
Lots of sex when drunk

(18-20)Abusive relationship (2 years)
Started cutting

(15) Parents Divorced / Binging Started

(10) Ate lots of candy alone when my dad was drinking

Figure 6.1 Timeline example

problem"), Safety/Vulnerability ("I am not safe, I cannot trust anyone") and Power/Control ("I'm powerless, I'm not in control"). If we listen to client descriptions and language of past events, we can often hear these distortions usually falling into one of the categories. Unprocessed trauma causes us to react to the present with the inadequately processed material of the past. Even if we are not formally trained in EMDR, identifying these themes can be extremely meaningful to highlight with clients and connect to current behaviors and symptoms (Shapiro, 2018).

When we are unable to process and integrate traumatic events, our bodies do the best they can to manage. Our bodies often become the canvas by which control, pain, shame, anger, and dysregulation are painted. Most trauma treatment experts catalogue eating disorders, addiction, and self-harm as an expression of the body related to safety, control, responsibility. It is mentioned in other chapters of this book that any traumatic event can affect sexuality and intimacy, not just trauma related to sexual abuse and assault. As we have explored thus far in this chapter, inadequately processed trauma generally impacts our ability to be present to our body, to regulate, and to care for it. Related to sexuality we find a myriad of difficulties expressed in basic functioning: desire, arousal, pain. Trauma is also expressed in difficulty regulating sexual behavior: excess masturbation or pornography use or sexual behavior with others to the point of interfering with health or daily living. Difficulties are also seen in problems experiencing and interpreting one's own body or communicating needs with others (Driscoll & Flanagan, 2016).

When we consider developing a treatment plan, reconnecting to the body's needs and messages is a key element of intervention. More will be discussed on these interventions in Chapter 11. Understanding why the disconnection occurred allows for grief/loss and remembrance and mourning which can also be identified as trauma processing.

I have referenced *the thread* as a way to conceptualize the weaving of the past to present. When clients begin healing and reconnecting to themselves and their bodies, they also need to develop a desired future template for many aspects of their lives. This includes some of the basic functioning like sleep and eating. It also includes more relational aspects such as support, finding pleasure in activities and others and also touch and intimacy.

The future template allows the opportunity to hope and imagine what can be possible. As mental health clinicians we can help clients bridge behaviors from where they are to where they want to be. The interventions and modalities we use in creating this bridge are expansive. As an example, I may utilize Intuitive Eating strategies to help an individual approach eating in a new way as they heal and move toward a future template of not restricting or over-eating. When an individual has difficulty negotiating sexual needs, I might help them script and role play the process, paying attention to what feels good, strange, uncomfortable. We would process these emotions to understand why they might be present. In this chapter we have explored some concrete ways to connect the present symptoms in the body with past trauma. The intervention section of this text will consider specific interventions for creating a bridge to healthy sexual functioning as a future template.

Common Presentations of Sexual Trauma

Hypersexuality

Experimentation and enthusiasm for sexual expression can be very healthy. Being sexual often, or thinking about sex often, is different from hypersexual or compulsive sexual behavior. Hypersexuality is behavior that is not directly related to pleasure. It sometimes results in the opposite of pleasure and feels like something that must be done versus something wanted or desired. This may occur in having sex with others many times a day, excessive amounts of masturbation or even high-risk sex. How do we objectively define excess? Listen for descriptions of the sexual behavior interfering with routine/time management, emotional distress or sometimes harm to body (e.g., soreness, chronic urinary tract infections). It is sometimes noticeable that there is a lack of explanation as to why the sexual behavior was being pursued. For instance, "I just had to have sex" or "I just kept masturbating even though I wanted to be done." The sexual behavior seems disconnected from a clear read on desire, interest or pleasure of the individual. We can also listen to distress or complications in relationships. This is often present with sexual partners who might be overwhelmed by the demand to be sexual.

The connection of past sexual abuse/assault and hypersexuality can be difficult for some to understand. It can be confusing why something that brought pain would become something done in excess. It seems it is an issue of lack of protection. Research on sexually compulsive behavior (as defined in ICD-11) or hypersexuality points to symptomatology as avoidance, re-experiences, and hyperarousal. It is very common for the individual to express regret, guilt, and shame related to the behavior. It seems that some part of the individual is pursuing a sexual pattern that another part of the individual is almost rejecting. Another way of conceptualizing this: the body is driven toward something and the intellect of the individual is not engaged or in agreement with it (Fontanesi et al., 2021).

When we look at the connection between past trauma and depression, we can understand the behavior as a stimulation or hyperarousal of the system that is craved. The repetitive pattern of the hypersexual behavior seems somewhat dissociative. It can be understood as a coping of shutting off or avoiding. Re-experiencing, like traumatized play in children, is an unintentional recreation of the trauma or some version of it, in an effort to make sense of it and eventually "work it out," or come to a new conclusion. For so many of my clients, I have noticed that even if their sexual choices are risky or without pleasure, they are in charge of the decision or at least determining that it will happen. This is a change in the narrative of their sexual story: I am doing it versus it is being done to me. I might not even like it but I decided it would happen (Fontanesi et al., 2021).

Hyposexuality

Sometimes clearer to the outsider looking in is the rejection or dislike of sexual behavior after experiencing sexual abuse/assault. There is often the connection of depression, guilt, and shame associated with trauma and a shut-down of emotions, connection, and even pleasure. The body often speaks for and protects the person in a way that sometimes they are not able or ready to do logically or verbally. A complete lack of sexual feeling or desire is not always but can be the body's expression of protection. It is a way of demonstrating, "I will not want what has brought me harm."

It is a common clinical presentation to have an individual who perhaps meets the diagnostic criteria for Female Sexual Desire/Arousal Disorder but does not initially discuss or label experiences in the past as trauma (although they were). Detailed assessment is so important to ensure we are developing an accurate narrative of the presenting problem so as to not "fix desire," when it is better understood as a protective reaction to past trauma. Helping the body feel again or want again is about helping the body, the person, heal the trauma.

Pain

Sexual pain is also commonly associated with experiences of sexual abuse or assault. Dyspareunia, a medical term for pain during intercourse, may be included during initial penetration of the vagina or pain with deeper penetration. Vaginismus is another type of pain disorder that is an involuntary contraction of vaginal muscles, blocking or making penetration of any form difficult. There can be an association with this type of pain and a history of trauma. It does not ignore other concerns that could lead to this condition such as childbirth or hormonal change due to menopause. As mentioned in earlier sections of this book, chronic pain can be connected with chronic trauma and chronic stress. When I hear clients discussing chronic health problems and chronic discomfort, I almost always suggest that their body is sharing a message. When clients can listen to this message it is amazing what they hear, "I need to slow down, I need time for myself, I've been neglecting myself, I'm hurt." I would encourage using this question, or a similar question, in your own work to help integrate body/mind insight with clients.

Degrees of Dissociation:

> Patterns of dissociation and avoidance can be common for sexual trauma survivors.
>
> Dissociation can best be understood as a coping mechanism along a continuum of severity. The Diagnostic and Statistical Manual of Mental Disorders defines three primary types of dissociation: Dissociative Identity Disorder, Dissociative Amnesia, Depersonalization/Derealization Disorder. These more severe presentations are described or specified as:
>
> Derealization, causing a feeling of distortion related to the world surrounding the individual. Simply described: "none of this feels real."
>
> Depersonalization, causing a feeling that the person themselves is not real in the form of disconnection from thoughts, sensations, feelings, identity.
>
> Dissociative Amnesia, when an individual reports knowing a traumatic event occurred but cannot remember the event in any detail or some aspects are not remembered
>
> Dissociative Identity Disorder, when the individual creates identities within themselves that are often triggered, switch, or become present related to stress, anxiety or fear.

It is important to understand that dissociation is not intentional, rather it serves to manage overwhelming circumstances. In many cases, the system or individual becomes "too good at it." On a mild level, any individual may temporarily avoid, "zone out" or daydream. More severe types of dissociation are often understood as a way for the system to be present, yet not present, in the face of something overwhelming to the system or something traumatizing (APA, 2022).

In the context of social work and sexuality, these terms are important to be aware of because dissociation serves to help the individual be less present, sometimes less aware of the trauma. However, the impact of the trauma still exists, often presenting in sensations, beliefs of self or others or illness/ dysfunction in the body. Difficulty being present in the moment, or in the body, because it wasn't safe in the past, often results in difficulties being present in sexual experiences. In the following chapters addressing treatment, we will offer tools to help the client safely become more present to moments and sensations (Pulverman & Meston, 2019).

The experience of trauma causes the human system to respond with coping mechanisms on a conscious and unconscious level. Addictive or compulsive behaviors are often viewed as a response to trauma. Author and Psychiatrist Bessel Van der Kolk believes that it is not possible for a behavior to become abused or addictive without the connection to trauma (Van der Kolk, 2014). Sometimes the "too much" or "too little" behaviors are directly expressed in sexual behavior resulting in "needing" or avoiding sexual experiences in a way that is not fully conscience or describable for the individual. Remaining curious about the behaviors is the first step in increasing insight. Other steps that may often apply:

- Being curious
- Exploring pattern
- Identifying emotional, somatic, cognitive triggers
- Labeling/Validating behavior as coping mechanism
- Identifying future template

Case Example

Client, Juan, 25 years of age, identifies as cisgender and gay. He has been in therapy for three months. He comes in for his session presenting low energy and "feeling down." He describes drinking too much last night and of course, "hooking up once again with the guy who doesn't treat him well." He remembers feeling "up-tight" early in the evening at the bar and has no idea how he got talked into going back to the guy's place.

The Therapist Responds

"I wonder if we can take a deep breath and try to release some of the feelings that are there for you right now, whatever they may be." (Takes deep breath with client)

He cries a bit.

Therapist:	I wonder if we could look a little more deeply into what might be happening for you when you end up doing something you actually don't want to do. Can we lay aside the idea that it is just a BAD decision and be curious about what might be directing you to this person or behavior?
Juan:	Yes, but it just feels so automatic.
Therapist:	Sometimes the things that feel automatic often have messaging from our environment, others' behaviors, expectations of our self that were written in our stories a long time ago. If we can become more aware of the messages, we can often be less automatic and challenge them.
Juan:	Okay, I can try.
Therapist:	So when you think back to last night it sounds like you didn't intend to have sex with this man at the beginning of the night? How were you feeling when you got to the bar?
Juan:	Pretty relaxed. I was meeting up with a couple good friends to hang out a bit. Danny (the guy he hooked up with) walked in and I remember thinking, oh here we go. See that's so stupid. I should have left right then.
Therapist:	So it sounds like there is a lot of judgement there. Why is it stupid? Why should you have left?
Juan:	I just hate that I always get talked into things I don't really want to do. I don't even know how it happens. It makes me feel weak and stupid.
Therapist:	Okay, so let's just take two or three steps away from the scene of last night and look from a distance at what is happening to Juan when Danny walks in and what is Danny doing?
Juan:	Me, I'm feeling up-tight when he walks in. I want to leave but something about Danny makes me feel like I owe him.
	Juan pauses for a bit and stares off.
Juan:	I think it is that I had sex with him before so it is unspoken, I just owe him again.
Therapist:	If you imagine that is not a rule you wrote but one you were taught, do you have any idea where you learned that rule… that you owe him because you had sex with him before?
	Juan begins to get very angry now. He is swearing and crying.
Juan:	I let myself get hurt, I let people do things to me and they always told me I liked it. I always thought it was something I did.

Therapist:	I'm so grateful you are unpacking this. You didn't make this rule. And this guilt and this thing that feels automatic, is something much deeper than that.
Juan:	I never make the rules. That's the problem. I never did. Danny does. My uncle did, my older cousin did.
Therapist:	When these things happened as a child the only thing your child self could do is believe the people who were supposed to be good and family. It makes so much sense that you would believe them.

In this case example, there are examples of several of the skills mentioned previously. Review the case study on your own or with a classmate and see if you can identify the different therapeutic skills of curiosity, exploring pattern, identifying emotional, somatic, cognitive triggers, labeling/validating behavior as coping mechanism

It important to remember that trauma that is unrelated to sexual abuse or assault also impacts sexuality and expression. There are several fields of research that highlight the multiple responses the body has on system regulation and connection and attachment. Unprocessed or unresolved trauma results in a body that is often operating in a sympathetic state or dorsal state, using the language of Polyvagal Theory. Polyvagal Theory is a theory based on three main neural states necessary for prosocial behavior and higher-level thinking. The sympathetic and dorsal states are key to mobilization (sympathetic), a reaction to danger in the form of fight flight and immobilization (dorsal) to survive when there is danger we cannot flee from.

The language of Polyvagal Theory helps us to understand that once again this is not occurring on a cognitive level but a way the system copes and constantly responds to a threat. These traumatic experiences may have been attachment injuries, early learned experiences threaded with emotional, physical abuse, neglect, lack of response, enmeshment. These traumatic experiences may have been related to bullying, witness to violence or systemic experiences of trauma such as discrimination. What links the experiences of trauma is that it places the human system in a place of survival response (fight/flight or sympathetic system), it alters opportunities to focus on the growing and developing relational nature of our human system and it becomes focused on intricate ways of surviving. When we consider trauma in clinical work, we need to consider the importance of processing what did occur (the awful/painful events) and what didn't occur because trauma was present (the growing, learning, play, connection, etc.). These experiences may not be directly related to sexuality. The limitations they place on human connection and the coping mechanisms that are developed to manage the trauma often limit our ability to be present and engaged. Being present and connected is required for intimacy (Dana, 2020).

The field of social work is continuously growing and changing. Trauma-informed treatment has been developed based on new understandings of how the body, mind, and spirit experience trauma. Several theories and modalities have helped us to understand the human processing of trauma. These theories help us construct and adapt the trauma narrative. This process allows us to make meaning of what has occurred. Trauma resiliency requires us to make meaning of what has occurred. Modalities associated with trauma-informed treatment include:

> Somatic Experiencing, developed by Peter Levine, is a bottom-up approach, meaning that information and focus starts with body sensations and moves toward cognitions. Increased awareness of the internal experience helps unlock trauma stored within the body. Clinicians focus the client on sensations, guide through imagery and interpret behavioral responses and affect to better understand the experience of the individual (Levine, 1999).

> Sensorimotor Therapy, created by Pat Ogden, is also a bottom-up approach that incorporates body awareness in clinical practice. Rather than cognitions, the body sensations are the focus. The clinician works with the client to target habits of physical action, autonomic dysregulation and posture to heal and inform change (Ogden, 2006).

> Eye Movement Desensitization Reprocessing (EMDR), developed by Francine Shapiro, focuses on changing the emotions, thoughts or behaviors resulting from a distressing issue. EMDR allows the brain to naturally continue the healing process. The use of dual attention stimulus and bilateral stimulation are used to process distressing or traumatizing memories resulting in decreased distress and new cognitions related to the memory and self (Shapiro, 2017).

> Polyvagal Theory, developed by Stephen Porges, focuses on education about and co-regulation of three primary neural states, ventral, sympathetic, and dorsal. It focuses on co-regulation of therapist and client as a neural exercise of prosocial behavior to develop self-regulation in a way that is often blocked by trauma experiences and chronic danger states (Dana, 2020).

> Internal Family Systems, developed by Richard Schwartz, is used for the treatment of most mental illnesses including trauma-related difficulties. Focused on the theory of multiplicity of the mind, IFS uses the language

of parts of self, to reach the goal of integration of parts and empower healing of the "Self," or entire system (Schwartz & Sweezy, 2020).

Questions to Prompt With/Topics to Cover

Let's assume that a biopsychosocial assessment has been completed and little information about difficulties with sexuality and intimacy was shared. As the trauma history is explored or as symptoms of past trauma in current functioning are identified, some of the following topics are important to cover:

Health and Wellness

From a biological perspective, chronic or complex trauma most often results in increased cortisol levels in the body and decreased effectiveness of the usefulness or messaging of cortisol over time. Disrupted eating patterns and sleeping patterns and inflammation in the body are common outcomes of the experience of ongoing trauma on the body.

Individuals who have faced one or multiple traumatic events that have not had the opportunity to heal often develop patterns of coping with symptoms that result in excess or deprivation of basic needs. Examples might include eating patterns, use of medications or self-medicating or even isolation versus socialization.

Questions to Prompt Conversation

Do you find it easy/difficult to care for the needs of your body on a daily basis?

Do you feel comfortable and able to speak with your medical doctor on an annual basis?

Do you find that you over-use/under-use food, sleep, medications, masturbation as way to respond to your body's needs?

Self-Care

Trauma held in the body most often serves to disconnect the individual from their body. A more direct way to explain this is that it can feel uncomfortable or painful to be aware of the body so, ignoring needs or dissociating on some level from body sensations is common. Hygiene problems and unaddressed physical or mental health symptoms are common for sufferers of chronic trauma.

Questions to Prompt Conversation

What are the main ways you take care of your physical, emotional, and spiritual health?

Do you find it difficult or overwhelming to know or respond to your body, mind, and emotions?

What has changed in your self-care?

Response to Body Sensations

Dissociating from the experiences of the body is a common way to keep one's self safe in a time of trauma. When triggered in the present by memories of the past, tuning out of one's body can become a coping mechanism of daily life. The body sensations we need to direct our attention to safety, wellness, care, and connection are often unavailable to sufferers of trauma.

Questions to Prompt Conversation

Are you able to receive signals from your body regarding need for sleep, hunger/fullness, need for closeness/affection?

Do you ever feel overwhelmed by certain body sensations? Can you describe that?

Trust and Closeness to Others

Most experiences of trauma affect the ability to trust one's self as well as others. The flood of cortisol, the neural pathways that are built on distrust and harm rather than trust and safety often result in poor boundaries, unspoken needs or sometimes isolation. A trauma experience means helping an individual regain trust in self, in others, as well as reading the spoken and unspoken messages to assess safety and navigate healthy boundaries.

Questions to Prompt Conversation

How have relationships changed for you since your traumatic experience?

What are your expectations of others in a close relationship?

How do you navigate consent and emotional/sexual boundaries in relationships?

Becoming a specialist in trauma-informed care truly requires additional training and supervision after graduate studies. To be prepared, informed, and prepared to ethically serve our clients upon graduation we must be able to conceptualize trauma. We need to be able to listen for and see its common and sometimes uncommon presentation in clients. The tools provided in this chapter will allow you to develop an informed case conceptualization of symptoms and the trauma narrative. This chapter has discussed directions of treatment when there is a history of sexual abuse/assault identified as well as directions of treatment when there are concerns of compulsivity, lack of feeling or pain without direct discussion of trauma. All traumatic experiences can cause distress in our bodies and stall healing. Awareness of what is blocked and hurt, as well as reflection and acknowledgement of trauma, are key to the healing process of trauma informed care. This chapter provides you with tools to begin that work. Good luck!

Questions for Reflection and Discussion

What limitations do you experience with thinking about trauma-informed care and sexuality? Do the limitations ever cause you to avoid discussion of the topic? What are ways you can address this?

What are ways that your own body responds when addressing trauma in a client session? How do you manage that in a session or after a session?

Diagnosis of Sexual Difficulties   **7**

Introduction

Diagnosis requires that we are able to hear specific symptoms within a client's presentation of problems. These symptoms lead us to specific criteria. Proper diagnosis leads us to intervention planning to address the presenting problems.

Presenting Topics/Problems of Sex Therapy

The Diagnostic and Statistical Manual (DSM-5-TR) provides diagnostic criteria for common symptoms and presenting issues of sex therapy. Sex therapists use the entirety of the DSM in their work when identifying and understanding presenting problems. Mental health professionals who have not sought additional training in sex therapy often have no experience utilizing the section of the DSM labeled Sexual Dysfunctions. As a result, underlying problems that influence presenting symptoms are often unrecognized and untreated. An example to demonstrate:

Case Example

Roger is a 55-year-old man who identifies as cis-gender and heterosexual. He is biracial, Black, and Mexican-American. He is seeking treatment for

DOI: 10.4324/9781003166382-8

symptoms related to mood disorder, consistent sad mood more days than not, decreased pleasure in most domains of his life, decreased energy, irritability, and anhedonia. He is employed in a career that he feels well-suited for and appreciates his coworkers. He has a good relationship with his adult son. His wife passed away after a long battle with cancer five years ago and he continues to miss her. He recognizes that he would like to have an intimate relationship in his life. Working diagnosis is Persistent Mood Disorder. Grief and loss issues are explored as part of treatment.

The mental health professional familiar with a sexual health assessment asks about his current relationship with his body, desire, pleasure, and masturbation. Gender identification, expression, and sexual orientation are also explored. Assessment includes questions about his past sexual experiences, use of fantasy, erotica, and pornography and description of ideal sexual experiences. Roger shares that he experienced difficulty with erections for the majority of his marriage. This difficulty has influenced not only the quality of his relationship but also his belief about himself. He noted that the guilt and shame he experienced caused him to isolate himself from his wife and diminished the quality of their relationship. He deeply regrets this disconnection. He fears entering a new relationship for similar reasons, although he craves the sexual connection and companionship.

The resulting material gathered through the questions regarding sexual health provides a much clearer picture of his mood disorder and the underlying factors. While the loss of his wife initially described is helpful in understanding his sadness, there is complexity to his grief. He holds regret and guilt related to the disconnection with his wife while she was still alive. There is also shame related to his sexual expression due to the chronic experience of erectile dysfunction. These factors also serve to inhibit moving forward in a relationship. The diagnosis may now be presented as Erectile Dysfunction with a secondary diagnosis of Persistent Mood Disorder.

When a mental health practitioner identifies as a sex therapist there is a higher likelihood that the presenting problem will include sex-related difficulties. Without that identification most clients need prompting to explore this domain of their lives and the expertise to connect sexual difficulties with other symptoms being reported.

Sexual dysfunctions may have a biological underpinning; however, there is always a contextual experience that is best explored through the intrapersonal, interpersonal, and cultural context of the individual. The diagnostic criteria of sexual dysfunction in the DSM-5-TR identifies symptoms qualifying as disordered that are woven in biological, sociocultural, and psychological factors. When there is sexual difficulty or dysfunction, and the source of the difficulty is better explained by a mental disorder, then the sexual dysfunction is considered a symptom of the primary diagnosis.

The DSM-5-TR identifies several disorders based on biological sex: Female Interest/Arousal Disorder, Female Orgasmic Disorder, Male Hypoactive Sexual Desire Disorder. The names of these disorders can be confusing and limiting, when working with gender non-binary and transgender clients. Several diagnoses, including Delayed Ejaculation, Erectile Dysfunction, Premature Ejaculation, are specific to the function of the anatomy. Clinical judgement is recommended when determining how these diagnoses may apply to gender-diverse persons. The authors of the DSM-5-TR provide an acknowledgement of the limitations of these diagnostic criteria as it relates to gender diversity. The DSM can be viewed as a document in continuous revision based on research and influenced by the culture it exists within.

There are noteworthy differences in diagnostic coding in The World Health Organization's International Classification of Diseases (ICD)-11. Desire and arousal as well as orgasmic dysfunctions are generalized versus specifically divided among anatomy identified as "female" and "male" as in DSM-5-TR. ICD-11 allows for the inclusion of sexual dysfunction when it represents independent focus of treatment even when it is caused by nonsexual medical disorder. The DSM-5-TR directs the diagnosis to the specific mental and health condition with sexual dysfunction a symptom of that other diagnosis (Reed et al., 2016).

Considerations for Diagnostic Criteria

Sexual Dysfunction requires the consistent consideration of two factors: Generalized/Situational and Lifelong/Acquired. Generalized or Situational factors ask us to assess if the symptom occurs in all situations or only in specific situations. This might be specific to solo or partnered experience, certain environmental factors and certain relational factors. Lifelong or acquired is a consideration of timeframe. When assessing this information, we are inquiring regarding a baseline and if the condition has ever been different or if there was a time the individual was symptom-free. Diagnosis is often detective work and this information allows us to collaboratively explore the context of the dysfunction.

Additional factors to inquire about as we work to determine the diagnosis:

> **Partner factors**: Does the partner(s) have a mental or medical diagnosis that impacts sexual intimacy? Are there limitations or difficulties that the partner experiences related to sexual intimacy?

Relationship factors: Is there any history of emotional, physical, sexual violence? What is communication like in the relationship? How does the relationship address consent and the navigation of intimacy?

Individual factors: Is there a history of developmental trauma, sexual abuse, physical abuse? Are there issues of body shame? What is the degree of differentiation?

Mental/medical diagnosis and treatment: Is there a history of psychiatric difficulties (i.e., mood, anxiety, psychosis)? Are there untreated medical concerns? Is there a history of chronic pain?

Stressors: Are there financial stressors? Is there a lack of time or privacy for relational or personal care? Is there external support for the couple/family?

Cultural and religious factors: What is the messaging in the culture and religion related to sexual expression? Are there specific sexual behaviors that are considered problematic or stigmatized?

Sexual Dysfunction Diagnosis

Delayed Ejaculation is defined as marked delay in ejaculation or infrequence or absence of ejaculation in 75–100% of occasions. There is not a specific timetable to reference related to how long average time to ejaculate may be in a solo or partnered experience. Research generally identified an average of four to ten minute range to reach ejaculation. This research is predominately based on penis and vagina penetration. Distress experienced by the individual and discomfort in the body of the individual and/or partner due to excessive thrusting are more useful symptoms than measurements of time in diagnosing this disorder.

A realistic clinical presentation of this disorder:

Stan is a 48-year-old bisexual, white man. He is seeking therapy related to low mood and mentions feelings of loneliness and isolation. He reports a key group of long-term friends but has not been in a relationship for almost a decade. In dating and intimate, sexual experiences of the last ten years, he has felt embarrassment related to the inability to orgasm or ejaculate. He describes excessive effort in thrusting and partner's judgement related to be "unable to finish."

Lifelong/*Acquired*: Stan reports he was able to orgasm and ejaculate in partnered sex with man and women earlier in his 20s and early 30s.

Generalized/*Situational*: Stan reports the ability to orgasm and ejaculate often during masturbation but not in any partnered penetrative sex, oral sex and partnered masturbation.

Brief Assessment: Relationship history reveals past history of partner shaming his body. Personal factors related to isolation and reliance on specific masturbation techniques (that cannot be duplicated with partners) have occurred in the last several years.

Erectile Disorder is defined as the difficulty obtaining an erection during sexual activity or difficulty maintaining an erection until completion of sexual activity or marked decrease in erectile rigidity. This occurs 75–100% of sexual occasions. Intermittent difficulty with erection duration or quality is expected over the lifespan and without duration of six months or more, should not be of concern. Medical problems such as diabetes and cardiovascular disease are often comorbid with erectile disorder. It is important to clarify expectations of duration as many individuals with a penis may hold expectations of endurance related to inaccurate depictions in pornography. Information about a recent experience and understanding the average duration of the erection, as well as how often this problem occurs and for how long, is important diagnostic information.

A realistic clinical presentation of this disorder:

Alejandro is a 25-year-old cisgender, heterosexual, Latinx man. He is married and has a young child with his wife. He reports concern that wife is interested in other men. He feels a sense of worthlessness. He describes his wife as critical of him. He feels worried and sad most days. He no longer enjoys being sexually intimate with his wife because he does not feel like he can please her. He often loses his erection within a few minutes of penetration. He reports feeling overly focused on his performance and concerned she is not pleasured.

> **Lifelong/*Acquired***: The problems with erection did not begin until the last six months when the concerns about infidelity began.
>
> **Generalized/*Situational***: Alejandro can maintain an erection during masturbation and also reports nocturnal erections. *This helps us rule out medical concerns because he does experience erections. It is always best practice to refer for medical exam because of the comorbidity with cardiovascular conditions and erectile dysfunction.

Brief assessment: The relationship factors with his wife seem to have a strong overlap with the symptoms of erectile difficulty. The concerns of infidelity also seem to contribute to low self-worth which can have an influence on sexual expression and confidence. The stressors in having a new child may also factor into the presentation of problems. Concerns related to a new baby and sleep are important to explore.

Female Orgasmic Disorder is defined by marked delay or infrequency of or absence of orgasm or reduced intensity of orgasmic sensations 75–100% of sexual activity for six months or more. This does not include situations when a mental illness, medical condition, lack of stimulation may be primary reason for lack of orgasm. It is also important to identify if clitoral stimulation may result in orgasm but not vaginal-only stimulation/penetration; likewise, that would not meet the criteria for the disorder. A more accurate description of this disorder would be Orgasmic Disorder for individuals with a vulva/vagina. Research informing this criterion considers issues of pelvic nerve damage, changes in hormones related to aging and issues of vaginal atrophy thus the specific identification with vulvas and vaginas related to orgasm. However, the connection of female with vulva/vagina is not necessary and harmful as a diagnosis to individuals that may identify as gender non-binary or transgender and have a vulva/vagina.

A realistic clinical presentation of this disorder:

Debra is a 30-year-old, cisgender, heterosexual, Black woman. She is in a monogamous relationship with a partner of six years. She reports experiencing arousal during sexual experiences with her partner. She feels sadness and disappointment as well as a sense of disconnection from her body due to the inability to reach an orgasm. She expresses that she often feels "close or a build-up" but has never orgasmed. She does not feel comfortable masturbating.

Lifelong/**Acquired**: She has never experienced an orgasm

Generalized/**Situational**: There has never been an experience that she has had an orgasm.

Brief assassment: Debra experiences a fair amount of anxiety in most parts of her relationship. She describes not feeling confident in a lot of areas and often seeking reassurance from her partner. Even though her partner has found ways to bring her pleasure, she often feels self-conscious and embarrassed by her body reactions to pleasure. This can be distracting. The lack of knowledge or exploration of her own body may also influence her overall discomfort and difficulty reaching orgasm.

Female Sexual Interest/Arousal Disorder is defined by lack of or reduced sexual interest/arousal manifested in absent/reduced interest in sexual activity, absent/reduced sexual erotic thoughts/fantasies, no/reduced initiation of sexual activity and not receptive to partner's initiation, absent/reduced sexual excitement/pleasure in 75–100% of sexual encounters, absent/

reduced sexual interest/arousal in response to any internal or external sexual/erotic cues, absent/reduced genital or non-genital sensations during sexual activity in 75–100% of sexual encounters. These symptoms have persisted for at least six months and are not better explained by a medication, substance or another mental disorder. It is crucial to pay close attention to the timeframe of symptoms as variance in desire due any variety of stressors and changes in life circumstances can influence changes in desire and interest. Identifying distress related to these symptoms for the individual, versus relational conflict related to sex, is especially important in diagnosis. This diagnosis considers difficulty related to desire as well as arousal. Consider information explored in Chapter 1 regarding the Human Sexual Response Cycle. The biopsychosocial experience of arousal may be reduced or completely lacking, related to the arousal phase, for an individual with this disorder. It is a particularly difficult diagnosis due to the risk of inappropriately diagnosing a mood or relational issue as a sexual dysfunction. Considerations mentioned at the top of the chapter regarding limitations of research and language of the DSM-5-TR and its application and impact on gender diverse individuals.

A realistic clinical presentation of this disorder:

Michelle is a 25-year-old who identifies as gender non-binary, is biracial (Black and Latinx), pansexual and in a partnered relationship. They report a loss of interest to think about erotic thoughts, engage in solo fantasy/masturbation or partnered activity. They report a deep attachment for their partner and note that their partner is still attractive to them, but they simply have no desire to engage in sexual experiences in the last year. They had hoped it was just a phase, but now feel distress related to how it affects the relationship as well as their sense of self.

> **Lifelong/*Acquired***: Michelle notes a distinct change in desire and engagement in sexual activities in the last year.
>
> ***Generalized*/Situational**: The lack of desire is in all scenarios, solo, and partnered.

Genito-Pelvic Pain/Penetration Disorder is the persistent or recurrent difficulties with vaginal penetration during intercourse, marked vulvovaginal or pelvic pain during vaginal intercourse or penetration attempts, marked fear or anxiety about pain in anticipation or during vaginal penetration, marked tensing or tightening of the pelvic floor muscles during attempted penetration. These symptoms persist for six months or more. There may be additional medical diagnosis such as endometriosis or lichen sclerosis as well as hormonal changes such as declining estrogen levels and postmenopausal pain. An experience(s) of pain during penetrative sexual activities can lead to the fear of future pain. Fear of pain can lead to avoidance of activities and create a cycle of pain, avoidance, and tensing of pelvic muscles along with increased anxiety.

A realistic clinical presentation of this disorder:

Alex is a 30-year-old, transgender man who is biracial (Black and White) and bisexual. He reports that although he experiences interest in being sexual with partners, he has not had a pain-free experience of penetration in the last eight months. He notes that he has developed fear and stress when attempting penetrative sexual experiences, as well as some avoidance. He notes that there was some vaginal dryness related to hormone therapy a year ago which was the initial experience of pain. Even with the use of lubrication to address dryness, the pain has persisted. He experiences both fear/anxiety as well as physical tensing and pain.

> **Lifelong/*Acquired***: Alex notes that prior to a year ago there were most penetrative experiences without pain. The association with penetrative experience and pain was both physical and emotional, noting fear and anxiety resulting in somatic reactions to the thought or attempt toward penetration.

> **Generalized/*Situational***: Alex notes that with the introduction of lubrication he can have solo experiences of penetration that are not associated with pain.

Male Hypoactive Sexual Desire Disorder is the persistently or recurrently deficient or absent sexual/erotic thoughts or fantasies and desire for sexual activity. The symptoms have persisted for six months or more and are accompanied by distress. It is important to differentiate from desire discrepancy with a partner or relational stressors and conflict that may lead to decrease sexual interest specific to the partner.

A realistic clinical presentation of the disorder:

Mark is a 20-year-old, cisgender, heterosexual, white man. He shares that he had two sexual relationships in his teenage years that were very fulfilling. He notes that he generally perceived himself as having a "healthy interest in sex." He shared that he used to masturbate daily and had sexual thoughts/fantasies throughout the day, on most days. In his junior year of college, he had a sexual experience and felt judged and humiliated by the woman's reaction to him. Although he has been able to move past this situation, he believes that the lack of erotic interest, thoughts, engagement in sexual behavior started at that time.

> *Lifelong/Acquired*: Mark notes that he previously had solo and partnered sexual experiences that were positive as well as regular erotic thoughts and fantasies.

> *Generalized/*Situational: Since the symptoms started, the lack of interest, desire, engagement in sexual behavior is in all areas including solo erotic thoughts or masturbation and he has not had thoughts or sexual interactions with others.

Premature (Early) Ejaculation is a persistent or recurrent pattern of ejaculation occurring during partnered sexual activity within approximately one minute following vaginal penetration and before the individual wishes the ejaculation to occur. This diagnosis can also pertain to other types of penetrative activity, but duration criteria do not currently exist. The symptoms are consistent over six months or more and associated with distress. Distress associated with expectations of duration is important to assess. Beliefs held by the sexual partner, as well as cultural beliefs, influence expectations the individual holds for themselves. Research focuses more on lifelong versus acquired premature ejaculation. Initial experiences of early ejaculation when individuals have their first sexual experiences are somewhat common and would not meet the diagnostic criteria unless the experiences continue beyond six months.

A realistic clinical presentation of the disorder:

Devin is a 25-year-old, cisgender, bisexual, white man in a partnered/open relationship. He has experienced difficulty with premature ejaculation since his first sexual experience when he was 15 years old. He experiences ejaculation almost immediately upon penetration of the anus or vagina. He also experiences early ejaculation with oral sex, however he can "last" slightly longer. He feels shame and failure related to this and it has a very negative impact on his relationship. He is able to masturbate for three to four minutes before ejaculating.

> *Lifelong/*Acquired: Devin has experienced this problem consistently since beginning sexual experiences.

> *Generalized/*Situational: He has a slightly different experience with masturbation but still feels he is ejaculating before he wishes to even in those solo experiences. The symptoms occur with all sexual experiences that are partnered.

Substance/Medication-Induced Sexual Dysfunction is the clinically significant disturbance in sexual function developed during or soon after substance intoxication or withdrawal or after exposure to or withdrawal from a medication. The substance/medication is capable of inducing dysfunction. The diagnosis requires specific coding related to substance use disorder present as well as the type of substance including, alcohol, opioid, sedative, hypnotic or anxiolytic, amphetamine or other stimulant, cocaine, other substance.

Realistic clinical presentation of disorder:

Kevin is a 25-year-old, cisgender, gay, biracial (white and Latinx) man. He has recently completed an intensive out-patient treatment program for cocaine addiction. His partnered sexual experiences were often associated with the use of cocaine. Upon withdrawal from the substance, he experiences lack of desire and difficulty having erotic thoughts or fantasies. He has also noticed significant change to the rigidity of erections. He realizes that cocaine dramatically changed his relationship with his own body and his sexual expression.

> **Lifelong/*Acquired***: Kevin experienced symptom-free sexual experiences prior to substance use therefore this is an acquired disorder.
>
> *Generalized/***Situational**: Since withdrawal from cocaine, Kevin has experienced symptoms throughout his day, in all experiences. Due to the lack of desire and arousal, assessment considers when he previously would have experienced desire/arousal, either solo or with others, and notes the symptoms are consistent in all experiences.

Through a series of questions, we are able to understand if the problem experienced is related to a lack of interest or arousal, a problem of performance or an experience of pain. In this assessment process we are also interested in understanding the expectations of self, body, and relationship that an individual holds. For many individuals who have diagnosed themselves with erectile dysfunction or orgasmic disorder we are able to uncover myths they hold about the body and offer education and normalization of the sexual experience. For instance, many individuals will source orgasmic disorder because they have never had an orgasm through vaginal penetration alone. Substantial research identifies that individuals with a vagina experience orgasm through just penetrative sex among only approximately 18% of the population. More individuals experience orgasm only through clitoral stimulation. Education about the body would rule out the diagnosis of orgasm disorder in these cases (Herbenick, 2018).

Primary and Secondary Diagnosis

Inherent in the biopsychosocial approach to sexual difficulty we know that underlying issues exist and that does not mean that the sexual dysfunction is not diagnosed. A good example of this is pain disorder with a personal history of trauma. It is often identified in the assessment process that past trauma has occurred when there is a presentation of pain during sexual experience. The individual may meet the criteria for Genito-Pelvic Pain Disorder and addressing the past trauma may be included in the treatment approach.

For example:

Pamela has a history of sexual assault. She meets criteria for posttraumatic stress disorder. During assessment she discloses that she is avoidant of sexual intimacy with her current partner because of fear of pain and a history of genital pain related to penetrative sex. Further assessment reveals diagnostic criteria for Genito-Pelvic Pain/Penetration Disorder is met. The primary diagnosis is the main focus of treatment.

Primary: PTSD

Secondary: Genito-Pelvic Pain Disorder

(Wincze & Weisberg, 2015)

Dysfunction Not Diagnosis

Common concerns that are often discussed when exploring relationship functioning or personal coping mechanisms, many related to difficulty in sexual behavior. Desire discrepancy is a commonly used phrase in the field of sex therapy as well as being referenced in popular culture. When clients discuss this, they often identify a variety of underlying sexual, communication struggles and relational dynamics that are at the root of the discrepancy. It is important to note that the increase in exploration of diagnosis through social media and Web-MD motivates clients to advocate and present this concern; however, it is not a diagnosis. We may include it as a symptom of a larger issue and certainly still evaluate change and incorporate interventions. This may present very differently on a case-to-case basis.

Case Example

Bella is diagnosed with a mood disorder. She notes desire discrepancy as a problem in her relationship that is causing sadness and resentment toward her partner. She states that the depressive state seems to numb her desire for sexual intimacy. She has a hard time communicating with her partner. It is not a reflection of him, rather an aspect of her Major Depressive Disorder. She feels frustrated that he is not more understanding and often pressures her to address this because it is having a negative impact on the relationship.

We can note low libido or decreased desire as a symptom that we track related to Major Depressive Disorder. We could incorporate an objective in treatment planning to address this symptom and relational challenge. Goal: client will identify emotional states and associated needs with support system. We would not diagnosis Female Interest/Arousal Disorder because the MDD is directly correlated with the lack of desire.

"Sex addiction" is also referred to as a diagnosis or presenting problem. Sex addiction is not a diagnosis in the DSM-5-TR and identified as Compulsive Sexual Behavior in the ICD-11 rather than an issue of addiction. Many individuals are referring to repetitive sexual behaviors that interfere with functioning in multiple domains. The term "sex addiction" has historically been used to pathologize certain sexual behavior. It is important to ask clients to describe the specific behaviors that they are referring to and assess:

1. Is this a problem for them or a problem defined by someone else in their life?
2. Does it feel outside of their control to stop the behavior?
3. Is it associated with distress of interfering with functioning, in one or more domains of their life?

Chapter 10 will offer additional information about problems related to compulsive or out of control sexual behavior (Kraus et al., 2018).

Aging and Sex

Most cultures, especially the United States culture, operate with a belief that individuals 50+ are no longer sexual. We don't depict images of sexual satisfaction and older adults in advertisements, movies, etc. Research illustrates that these beliefs influence medical discussion and intervention, or lack thereof, between medical professionals and patients. Ideally medical professionals and mental health professionals would incorporate sexual health across the lifespan. Caring for and protecting one's body, protection, safety, consent, and pleasure should all be regular topics with clients and patients. Professionals should also discuss the natural ways the body changes with aging and how this may change sexual experiences.

Changes across the lifespan are researched and categorized based on biological male and biological female bodies. Changes in the neurology, nervous system, cardiovascular system as well as hormonal changes affect all bodies over the course of the lifetime, resulting in changes to the sexual experience. Changes over time impact experiences of desire and arousal. Individuals with a penis most often experience erectile difficulties or hypogonadism. Problems are associated with numerous factors including vascular disease, prostatic surgery/disease, diabetes, and the side effects of medications. Individuals with a vagina/vulva are more likely to experience difficulties in psychosocial factors, urogenital atrophy, urinary incontinence, and cancers that will affect sexual experience.

When we raise the topic of sexuality and functioning with older adults, we acknowledge part of their lived experience and relay a sense of understanding and respect. For some generations the topic may feel surprising and that does not mean that our questions are inappropriate, it means the experience is new. As mentioned in earlier chapters, associating sexuality with domains of health and functioning as is the rest of the topics of our biopsychosocial assessment is an ideal response and way to move forward (Taylor & Gosney, 2011).

Raising this topic can also offer new ideas to explore intimacy. Penetrative sex often becomes more difficult, and for some, less comfortable in later years of life. A few areas of importance to cover in the area of diagnosis, sexuality, and aging:

Expectations of Body

As mentioned previously, there are predictable changes that occur to the body over the course of the lifespan. These changes will influence erection, lubrication, tissue lining, and endurance. Normalizing changes and helping to adapt to them in a way that feels healthy for the body, and still allows for pleasure, is important. As an example: "you have a different type of erection versus an erectile dysfunction."

Changes, Not an End

Due to discomfort raising the topics in relationships and with medical or mental health professionals, misinformation is prevalent for aging individuals.

Opening the conversation with comfort and directness is crucial. Encouraging discussion of how their body is changing and what expectations they hold for sexual experiences is important. Sexual pleasure is completely possible but expectations must align and often be redefined in accordance with body changes.

Questions to Prompt Conversation

Are you currently enjoying sexual experiences?

Are there changes with your body that you have noticed influencing your sexual experience?

How are you navigating sexual pleasure (with self/partner) and changes to your body?

Conclusion

It is important to acknowledge that this overview of sexual dysfunction diagnosis' may be quite overwhelming. While you cannot consider yourself an expert, familiarity with terminology and symptoms will allow you to recognize problems and ask useful questions. Supervision in diagnosis is important as we begin our careers. Continued research and reading and clinical experience will move diagnostic ability from exposure and familiarity to expertise. Helping clients to name a difficulty often reduces shame and helps them enter a path toward intervention and solutions.

Questions for Reflection and Discussion

What implications and benefits exist for using the language of diagnosis related to sexual functioning?

Is there a specific diagnosis discussed in this chapter that seems problematic to you? Why? Would it cause you to avoid applying the diagnosis?

Guiding Clients to Good Enough Intimacy, Medical Difficulties/Diagnosis, Disabilities, and Sexuality

8

Introduction

Utilizing the biopsychosocial approach to assessment, we gather information about client's medical history and presenting concerns. Health problems and medications are important to understand, related to client's mental health, self-care, daily stressors, and responsibilities. Serious health conditions, chronic health problems, and physical disabilities often become the prominent concern of health providers, partners, and family members. It is important that we understand these challenges, related to the interplay of physical, mental, and socio-emotional well-being. Our treatment approaches will often focus not on alleviating pain or illness but on improving quality of life. While medical providers and family may have a hyper-focus on managing illness, mental healthcare expands the focus to other important aspects of the client's life. Mental health clinicians can place focus on intimacy and relationships that can sometimes be overlooked when illness is viewed as a large challenge.

Common Health Concerns

Any illness, severity or duration not-withstanding has an impact on other domains of functioning. More common issues such as urinary tract infections

DOI: 10.4324/9781003166382-9

(UTIs) and yeast infections can lead to negative consequences related to physical discomfort or decreased confidence. Chronic health problems may have a direct and indirect impact on sexuality and experiences of intimacy. It is helpful to have a broad understanding of how illness influences relationships and sexual functioning. This overview is certainly not an exhaustive list of chronic conditions but offers insight into effects we can prepare for as we approach assessment and treatment planning.

Cardio-Vascular Conditions

The biological experience related to sexual behavior, specifically that relying on genitals, relies on multiple systems of the body. Problems related to the vascular system often affect sexual functioning. Many chronic health problems impact blood vessels and blood flow. The Human Sexual Response Cycle includes increased blood flow that leads to enlargement of the nipples, clitoris, labia, and penis. Vasocongestion also results in uterine elevation (tenting). Narrowing of blood vessels, or problems with blood flow, inhibits this biological arousal process. This results in problems obtaining or maintaining erection of the penis and decreasing vaginal lubrication or vaginal elongation and vulvar/clitoral swelling. Sexual pleasure can be greatly reduced as a result of these difficulties with the arousal cycle. Sexual functioning making penetrative sex possible is also affected. Artery disease limits blood flow from the heart and causes narrowing of blood vessels. Diseases and conditions that lead to artery disease include high blood pressure, diabetes, high cholesterol, obesity, heart disease, coronary artery disease, and smoking (Foley, Kope, Sugrue, 2012).

Cancer

All types of cancer are generally associated with difficult treatments that may include chemotherapy, radiation, and surgery. Fatigue, loss of appetite, changes to body/appearance, scarring, weight loss, as well as emotional symptoms of grief, fear, isolation, and sadness are all common to cancer treatment. Both the emotional strain of cancer treatment as well as the treatment approaches themselves can impact sexual functioning.

Specific cancers such as breast, ovarian, uterine, testicular, and prostate can be especially detrimental to sexual functioning. Complications due to hormone treatment can result in forced and immediate menopause, changes to arousal, lubrication, and vaginal elasticity, vaginal atrophy. Hormonal treatments can also lead to development of male breasts, genital shrinkage, and erectile dysfunction. Significant grief and loss are associated with changes to body image with removal of body parts as well as secondary symptoms such as scarring, weight loss/gain, and changes to quality of skin.

Dermatological Conditions

There are several dermatological conditions that impact individuals due to discomfort, itching or decreased confidence due to appearance. Specific dermatological conditions can affect the genitals specifically. Hidradenitis Supertiva (HS) is a chronic, dermatological condition causing large lumps similar to boils, on the buttocks, armpits, breasts, and genitals. Pain, leakage, and odor are common. Medication and surgery may result in secondary symptoms impacting sexual function. Lichen Sclerosus is a long-term dermatological condition affecting genital and anal areas. It can make the skin thin, white, wrinkled, itchy, irritated, and painful. A similar condition and Lichen Planus can cause specific damage to tissue that is mucous membranes. Psoriasis can affect the genitals, specifically causing painful lesions.

Diabetes

Both type 1 and type 2 diabetes can have a harsh impact on the body and sexual functioning. Complications related to diabetes can include neuropathy, hormonal imbalances, and artery disease. Circulation problems may lead to significant difficulties with erection, lubrication, and decreased sensation in the genitals during sexual experiences. Vaginal dryness and increased yeast infections are also common health concerns for individuals with diabetes.

Auto-Immune

There are multiple auto-immune diseases including, Rheumatoid Arthritis, Lupus, Inflammatory Bowel Disease, Multiple Sclerosis, Guillain-Barre Syndrome, Diabetis mellitus (type 1), Chronic Inflammatory Demyelinating Polyneuropathy, Psoriasis, Graves Disease, Hashimoto's thyroiditis, Myasthenia gravis, Scleroderma, Vasculitis. Extreme low activity and low energy level is common with auto-immune conditions. The diseases attack joints, major organs, and muscle systems. Medication to suppress the immune system is the most common treatment. Due to the variety of presentations of these conditions it is difficult to pinpoint specific challenges to sexual functioning. Changes to quality of life and ability to function influence the level of energy individuals can offer to sexual relationships. Specific challenges related to nerve damage and muscle spasms can affect the arousal phase of sexual response resulting in difficulty with vasocongestion, lubrication, and erection.

Mental Illness

Mental illnesses and the medical treatment of mental illnesses can have a profound impact on sexual health and function. As discussed in Chapter 7, sexual problems are often comorbid with mental disorders (Southall & Combes, 2020). Broadly, we can consider how mental illness may impact energy, self-care, regulation, mood, and connection with others. The treatment of mental illness through medication may also have side effects that affect sexual function.

Anxiety Disorders and Somatic Disorders

Generalized Anxiety and Social Phobia can limit an individual's ability to be present to themselves and with others. Difficulty focusing, rumination, excessive worry can keep an individual from entering into desire or distract them from staying in that space.

Obsessive Compulsive Disorder

Similar to anxiety symptoms, OCD fixates thoughts away from desire and pleasure. Intrusive thoughts interfere in key relational capacity and certainly from sexual expression. Additionally, obsessions specific to cleanliness or sexually taboo thoughts can directly interfere with the feeling of safety and sexual behavior (Gordon, 2002).

Major Depressive Disorder

Depressive symptoms tend to "slow" the individuals in every domain. The lowered mood and lowered energy often pull them away from relationships, self-care, and participation in once-pleasurable activity. The depressed mood drastically decreases or completely mutes sexual desire (Kendurkar & Brinder, 2008).

Bipolar Disorders (1 and 2)

Individuals with bipolar disorder will experience major depressive episodes, decreasing the feeling of pleasure and desire for sexual experiences. Manic episodes, occurring with Bipolar 2, frequently result in high-risk sexual behaviors and poor decision-making that is uncharacteristic of the individual. The cycling of bipolar disorder, especially bipolar 2, can be consequential for stability in long-term relationships.

Eating Disorders

The underlying experience of anorexia nervosa and bulimia nervosa influence the relationship with sexual functioning. Individuals with anorexia experience an intense need to control the body. The symptoms of anorexia result in significant weight loss and fixation on food and weight. There is room for little else in terms of thinking or engagement beyond this. The individual with bulimia experiences consistent dysregulation in most domains of functioning. This includes the binge/purge of food as well as common struggles with relationships and mood. Dysregulation and fluctuation will often be seen in sexual behaviors and relationships (Castellini et al., 2012).

Personality Disorders

It is still sometimes debated whether severe attachment injuries are associated with the development of personality disorders; for those clinicians working from an attachment lens, it feels obvious. Individuals that have a diagnosed personality disorder will struggle with intimate relationships for different reasons.

Obsessive-compulsive personality disorder is defined by inflexibility, fixation with rules, and perfectionistic behaviors. If they are able to maintain relationships these problems will generally interrupt sexual pleasure with a fixation on perfection and rumination on the sexual process.

Narcissistic Personality disorder is best understood as a puffer fish, blown-up out of fear or neediness but feeling small and empty inside. The neediness and seeking validation make relationships unfulfilling and difficult to maintain. The difficulty to look into one's own responsibility and emotions offers significant challenges to the experience of all types of intimacy.

Borderline Personality Disorder is characterized by dysregulation of emotions and relationships. The push and pull of individuals they are in relationship with is experienced as exhausting and toxic for partners and support systems. Sexual relationships may be excessively pursued but often unstable or unfulfilling.

Avoidant Personality Disorder causes extreme difficulty in building relationships and socializing. Most often, if individuals are able to make a connection, they are able to feel fulfilled in caring relationships. Shyness and inhibition make sexual expression and connection extremely difficult.

Antisocial Personality Disorder is characterized by manipulative and exploitive behavior. These individuals often have more sexual experiences that are often based in toxic behavior and infidelity in relationships (Reise & Wright, 1996).

Neurodevelopmental Disorders

Attention Deficit Hyperactivity Disorder (ADHD), Learning Disabilities (LD) and Autism Spectrum Disorder (ASD) create significant challenges for individuals related to interpreting social cues and communication. Touch and the experience of bodily fluids in sexual experiences can be specifically difficult for some individuals with ASD. It is common for partners to be placed in care-giving roles as a way to help individuals with neurodevelopmental disorders manage daily routines. This relational dynamic can be burdensome in the long-term and have negative effect on sexual desire (Betchen, 2003).

Antidepressants, antipsychotics, and benzodiazepines used to treat depression, anxiety, and severe mental illness such as bipolar, schizophrenia or schizoaffective disorders may cause lack of or decreased desire, difficulty with orgasm, difficulty obtaining/maintaining erection, and painful sex. It can be extremely difficult to identify the source of the irritability, sadness, and disconnection reported by clients. Often it is not the disorder itself but the effect of the medication and the reduction in relational and sexual health that is the source of difficulty. Assessing the difficulties and close communication with the prescribing medical professional may allow for changing dose of medication, switching to another agent, or in some cases a "drug holiday."

Drug holidays are sometimes discussed with clients, when safe to do so, to allow for opportunities for positive sexual experiences without the influence of medication. These drug holidays acknowledge the problems with the medication, as well as the necessity of the medication, thus a holiday versus completely stopping the medication. Drug holidays are negotiated with a mental health professional, well-planned and short-term to allow for positive sexual experiences without the influence of the medication. They should be done in coordination with communication with prescribing doctor (Gitlin, 1994).

Neurological Conditions

Common neurological conditions include Parkinson's disease, multiple sclerosis, spinal cord lesions, epilepsy, and other types of seizures, traumatic brain injury and stroke. Any condition that affects the brain or nervous system will likely have affect sexual functioning. Individuals with Parkinson's disease often face especially difficult sexual effects including vaginal atrophy, decreased lubrication, incontinence, delayed ejaculation, and erectile dysfunction. Medication for Parkinson's, a dopamine agonist, can cause hypersexual desire and thus complications in partnered sexual relationship. Treatment for epilepsy is also associated with anorgasmia and decreased desire.

Assessing the Relationship of Physical, Relational, and Sexual Health

Given this overview of common illnesses that have significant impact on sexual functioning, we can be more prepared for assessment. During this initial assessment phase, information about the client's medical diagnosis, treatment, medication, and treatment side effects, and symptoms is shared. The following questions can be explored to gain more information about the socio-emotional and relational effect of the illness.

Understanding the Relationship of Illness and Body Image

Do you perceive your body differently since your diagnosis or pain/ symptoms started?

Does your illness/disease/pain have a direct impact on any part of your body?

How does your illness/disease/pain influence your belief about your body?

The Relationship of Illness and Socio-Emotional Health

How has the diagnosis changed your life?

How does it impact daily functioning?

How does the health issue impact your relationships?

How does your health issue limit favorite activities, hobbies?

How do you experience pain?

How does pain impact your energy?

Do you feel an increased desire to connect (seek comfort) or solitude when you are experiencing pain?

Does your illness/disease/pain require additional energy and attention that was previously directed at self-care or relationships?

The Relationship of Illness and Sex and Intimacy

How does your medication, treatment, pain impact your sexual experiences, partnered or solo?

Have you noticed a change in your interest in sexual pleasure or shared intimacy since symptoms started?

Are there parts of your body that you feel uncomfortable touching/ being touched or seeing/being seen?

These questions do not necessarily need to be asked in this order, or in totality, but a combination of the questions may help to acknowledge the connection between illness and sexuality. This can allow for a deeper understanding of the influence of illness. Often clients receive messages that their sexuality is not of primary importance when a serious health problem is being addressed. In a recent study of patients treated for bipolar disorder and sexual quality of life authors summarized, "taking the effects of mood treatment on SF [sexual function] into consideration would help improve treatment compliance and decrease lifetime suicide attempts and consequently optimize the quality of life of BD patients" (García-Blanco et al., 2020).

Major Themes

Relevant themes will surface when clients have the opportunity to consider the emotional, sexual, and relational implications of their illness. The basic act of identifying or naming the experience is, in and of itself, a treatment task. Identifying and naming ends avoidance and the underlying anxiety that comes with avoidance. The act of identifying and naming also allows for acknowledgement of the experience, as another person bears witness. Begin with this part of healing with the client and do not underestimate its importance. More specific themes that surface related to illness follow.

> *Grief:* One of the most common themes is grief. Grief and illness present in a number of forms. Grief for a way of feeling or presenting that is now gone. Grief for living with a sense of ease (without illness) that you perceive others around you are able to live. Grief for specific parts of life you have never or cannot experience. Grief about who you wish to be, that you cannot be. When you are working to survive or others are working to care for you, attention to the grief rarely occurs. Grief, unacknowledged or unprocessed, can cause isolation, lead to depression, reduce energy, and inhibit the immune system.

Cognitive Behavioral Therapy (CBT) is the most common approach in grief counseling. Asking the client to explain recent moments that grief is prominent and helping them develop insight into the negative patterns is a good place to begin in treatment. Psychoeducation related to grief as a cycle versus a linear process is important. Often clients will identify a sense of failure as they cycle through stages. Helping them identify their stages and view this as a process that holds information and insigIt is an important element of empowerment. The use of Internal Family Systems (IFS) to identify manager parts and protective parts that are helping them deal with grief, is a shift in thinking for clients. Rather than viewing thoughts and coping mechanisms as maladaptive, we can help clients develop compassion for the ways that parts are helping them manage. We also use IFS to explore the needs of support to develop increased self-communication and relational support.

Most of the problems clients face are not things that we can completely resolve; rather, we help them think differently about them or develop new strategies for living with or around the difficulty. Illness and sexuality are much the same. Sometimes injury, muscle spasms, damage to tissue, or surgery may make penetrative sex completely out of the question. When we help clients think about what they can do versus what they can't do, we help them identify solutions, or at least ideas that we can expand. Always allow for grief in the treatment process first. Seeking solutions will be met with resistance when grief is ignored.

Once we have acknowledged and validated the grief and loss associated with illness, clients are well-prepared to think about what is possible. If you find that clients avoid brainstorming solutions or reject ideas you propose, stop. Go back to the grief treatment interventions. I remind clients that our biggest sexual organ is our brains. We can be sexual in any way we wish to be. Specific approaches will be discussed in Chapter 11.

> *Body image*: Changes to body and lack of confidence about body image is a major experience of many illnesses. The ideals of body that are promoted in social media and pop-culture make it extremely difficult for individuals with chronic illness to recognize themselves. Certainly, images of individuals with chronic illness are almost never represented as sexual. Sometimes individuals will avoid using health aids or being consistent with medications or dietary restrictions in order to present closer to the "ideal."

> *Challenging*: Helping clients discover new images and models of beautiful and sexy within the community of chronic illness survivors is very important. National and local support groups as well as YouTube channels often offer alternative voices and images to the mainstream subscription of beautiful or sexy that includes chronic illness survivors and disabled bodies.

More specifically, reframing or challenging can be used to address parts of the body. Asking the client, "what is the story you tell yourself about that part of your body?" is a way to prompt this exploration. Similar to the following case study about Amanda, we can also challenge the script a client holds about the way others view their body. This can be done by encouraging questions/conversations directly with these other individuals or asking the client to journal a dialogue between themselves and the other person. The therapist can work with the client to challenge some of the assumptions noted within the dialogue.

> *Redirecting*: Moving mental energy and focus is a useful approach. Redirecting can be specific to sexual experiences. This technique is

addressed in detail in Chapter 11. Redirecting can also be used to place general focus and attention to other areas of the body. Self-care routines and highlighting other areas of the body such as weightlifting, coloring hair, getting nails done, can move focus a part of the body that they identify as "broken" or ill towards a part of the body they view in a positive manner.

I will use a case example to demonstrate these treatment perspectives:

Amanda is a 32-year-old, white, cisgender, heterosexual woman. She is married to Dan and they have a 4-year-old child together. Amanda was diagnosed with Hidradenitis Suppurative (HS) two years ago. The chronic inflammatory skin condition has caused several large lumps on her vulva. In addition to the pain, Amanda is very embarrassed by the condition. Her husband Dan is very supportive and expresses interest in sexual intimacy, but Amanda often feels ashamed of her body. She expresses that she cannot imagine Dan could actually be attracted to her with this condition.

(Grief) Amanda often felt resentful of friends or even strangers on social media that didn't have the illness. She had a hard time seeing the things that were going well in her life because she felt focused on the illness, despite trying hard not to think about it. She felt like a person she no longer recognized. Amanda had an entire treatment team, but most of the time they were focused on measuring, medicating, and even surgically removing the lumps. She needed permission to feel the grief. When she was able to make space for the grief, she gave herself permission to have those feelings. She also learned how to compartmentalize grief from other parts of her life. Being able to share the difficulties of her illness with her support system also helped to process the resentment that came with the grief.

(Body image) Amanda had surgery to her labia to remove a large lump. In addition to the scarring, she had additional lumps that had surfaced on her vulva. She noted that not feeling sexy directly caused a decrease in sexual desire. She also struggled with fear about allowing her partner to see her vulva. Her partner expressed a great deal of desire to touch her and have oral sex with her, but she avoided this because of the fear.

(Redirecting) When there is a body part that has changed and we have difficulty accepting the change, we can become hyper-focused on its importance or the image we hold of it in our mind. At the end of one of our early therapy sessions I asked her to talk to her husband about his experience. What does he enjoy about having oral sex with you? Ask him to describe what the experience is like for him. When she returned for the next session, her attitude felt noticeably lighter. She shared with me that her husband described several amazing sensations he experiences about having oral sex with her.

Hearing his description was reassuring and helped her understand her body and the experience from his perspective. This also helped her walk back from her hyperfocus on a very negative image she had created in her mind.

Amanda's pain on her vulva due to the surgery scars and new lump were significant. Her partner would snuggle up for a kiss and she would feel sad and dismiss his attempts. She felt like intimacy would lead to sex and she was fearful of penetration. We talked about "No. . .but" as a strategy. Amanda thought about the things she does like to do with her partner like cuddling, massaging, and even making out on the sofa. The next time her partner approached her she said, "no I can't have sex, but I would love to kiss on the couch." She even got better at initiating these encounters and felt empowered by the practice.

Disability

The topic of disability includes physical, developmental, emotional, and sensory-impaired. Experiences of disabilities are diverse. Individuals with acquired versus congenital disabilities will have differing journeys with grief, acceptance, and adjustment. Often, disabled individuals are seen as asexual and treated as such. The space of therapy to recognize them as a sexual person is often validating but may also be extremely vulnerable, possibly overwhelming, scary or uncomfortable. It is important to help them think about,

> How they would like to be seen as a sexual person?
>
> What they would like to experience sexually?

The treatment issues that have been discussed to this point related to chronic illness can very well apply to disability individuals. Grief for ways that their body and experience is different from others and loss for experiences they did not have or may have lost access to is very important to identify. Increasing access to images of disabled bodies and voices of disabled educators and activists may also be very useful. Combating messages about what is not available or what they cannot be is imperative.

The research points to the common problem of disabled individuals not having access to sex education and opportunities because they are too often viewed as asexual. An important social justice issue in the disabled community is the right to be treated as a sexual person, education about sex and their bodies and sex facilitation. Dependent on the disability, a person may need assistance being sexual either solo or partnered. Often parents or care providers view this as inappropriate or outside the scope of care rather than view this as a sexual right. Rather than continuing this injustice we have the opportunity to explore how someone would like to be sexual, provide education about body and emotional safety and provide planning ideas for facilitation.

Assisting with facilitation for sex may include access to devices and props that allow individuals to access their bodies or position their bodies in ways to be sexual. Access may be about helping them have conversations with family or care staff about their sexual rights. Access may also be about planning for safe ways to be sexual with boundaries and expectations.

In the case of developmental disabilities, we can recognize the importance of describing sex education concepts in a way that is approachable. We may also want to ensure the rules and expectations held by people they are living with or are being cared for by are encompass and sex positive. Offering approachable sex education to family and care staff can also be very useful. The hard limit of "no" that is often used to govern disabled individuals from sex is not only unjust, it results in a much higher degree of sexual abuse occurring to this population than the general population. Exceptional resources exist for providing sex education and creating plans for safe sexual exploration.

Making space for the recognition of each individual client as a sexual person is important to our work in social work and any mental health profession. When people are denied or do not have resources for safe intimacy and exploration of their own selves or in connection with others, they are harmed. Processing grief and loss paves the path for acceptance and the development of new ways of meeting sexual and socio-emotional needs.

Chronic illness, mental illness, and disabilities change the experience of sexuality. It is important for mental health practitioners to understand and inquire about the specific ways that sexuality may be affected. Adaption and resources to find new ways to be sexual is possible and an important part of well-being.

Questions for Reflection and Discussion

Why does sex seem like an extra or a bonus or even inappropriate when individuals are addressing serious illness or have a disability?

If you were working with an individual with a cognitive disability, what fears would you have for advocating for their sexual expression?

Stigma, Societal Messages and Sexual Difficulty

9

Introduction

Articles and discussions about pleasure often begin by attempting to define sexual pleasure and quickly morph into the specific techniques to acquire pleasure. This can become difficult to maintain the concept of sexual pleasure as completely unique to the person while still offering specific suggestions on what might help someone increase pleasure. Sexual pleasure is also a multi-billion-dollar industry complete with magazine articles, toys, and props, pornography, medication, and even surgeries. Helping individuals remain grounded in sexual exploration that is unique to them, and not fixated on improving performance, is important and difficult.

Sexual performance relies on a standard of how the body should respond. It encourages measurement of pleasure in comparison to a standard, a norm, others, versus pleasure as a unique experience. The language of performance asks: Am I hard enough? Did I last long enough? Is it big enough? Did he/she/they cum? Was I wet enough? Was I tight enough? The language of pleasure asks: Did I feel emotionally engaged? Did my body feel open and responsive to what was happening? Did my body respond in readiness? Beyond pleasure, we can also evaluate sexual experiences related to comfort, curiosity, connection, and learning.

Challenging Myths and Unhealthy Expectations

As sex educators and therapists there is a noticeable change in sexual information and expectations based on generational influence. Baby Boomers

DOI: 10.4324/9781003166382-10

and Generation X did not come of age in a society that offered the benefit of immediate access to diverse information. To speak in generalities for a moment, it is less common for clients in these generations to have conducted the same level of internet "research" as the Millennials and Gen Z/igen generations. There are pros and cons for all the generations. Having information readily available, from multiple sources, often allows individuals to have a basic level of preparedness, related to safety and health. This is of course influenced by browser history and the direction the user chooses to go on the Internet. Often, the information can be misleading or confusing.

Assessment and psychoeducation should include understanding primary sources from the internet and offering some reliable spaces for information. The increased reliance on the internet generally allows people to be more familiar with information related to sexuality. Familiarity with terms and concepts may result in clients feeling more confident in discussing topics. Recognizing the generational differences in accessing information and its influence on comfort with the topic of sexuality is important. Recognizing that clients will have differences in how they access information allows us to prepare resources in a diversity of styles. As you build your resource library on topics of mental health, self-care, and sexuality, consider having at least one book, one article, one video and a form of social media that can be provided for each topic.

The internet also made pornography instantly accessible. Due to the unbelievably limited sex education offered in most school systems, and the continued difficulty parents/guardians often experience discussing sexuality and intimacy in approachable ways with youth, pornography often serves as the primary tool of young people use to learn about sex. Consuming pornography can be beneficial for individuals to explore their sexual interests; however, it is imperative that it is understood as fantasy and not a form of sexual education. The harm perhaps is not pornography, or access to pornography, rather the lack of conversation and education from real folks in teen's lives to make sense of and balance the messaging in porn.

Pornography is often reported as a problem in family work or couples work because of the type of pornography that is being viewed. Psychoeducation related to pornography as a form of fantasy is very important. Certainly, individuals may name cultural, religious, and ethical reasons they find pornography problematic. The concern that someone wants sex that is "like the porn" often surfaces. Most fantasy deviates from what we need/ want in daily life. Fantasy offers a release from the expectations we hold of ourselves and others in reality and allows us to "play" by stepping outside of our rules. Helping individuals explore this, rather than setting behavior rules or expectations surrounding use of pornography, is beneficial.

Online dating has greatly influenced the language, expectations, and norms of sexual engagement. Depending on the dating app, the behavior required is more performative and transactional and less relational. Online dating can be especially hard for individuals with limited confidence. Navigating this environment is often a topic in therapy. We can be of most benefit to clients when we help them think about what they are seeking and how they communicate that message. The measurement of swipe left versus swipe right can create a highly performance-focused marketplace of negotiating relationships. "Matching" can feel like a win or a triumph. Similar to dating in-person, an individual can be reduced to the image they present, and a series of behaviors that pass a test and wins attention. I encourage clients to stay grounded in what they are seeking, e.g., a relationship, a friendship, a sexual interaction, and negotiate that directly. Risk and regrets can be minimized by discussing expectations before meeting in-person. Caution is advised related to exploring a brand-new sexual behavior with a brand-new person. At minimum, it is helpful to help the individual consider what they expect from pleasure or discomfort in the experience and what risks are associated.

As clinicians we begin by assessing the messages clients were handed and those that they would like to keep and those they need to discard. Sex educator, author, and researcher Emily Nagoski uses the metaphor of a garden with messages we weed out, new concepts, and beliefs we plant (Nagoski, 2015). As adults, we have the choice to accept/continue the societal, religious, family, and peer messages we received growing up and we empower our clients to embrace this same choice and responsibility. The sexual health assessment offers questions to help clients reflect on the implicit and explicit sexual messaging in their history. Our learning is layered and often based on the nonverbal and is based in attachment-informed reactions and body reactions. Questions that focus on "What do you remember?" and "What meaning did you make of that?" allow clients to rely on their implicit knowledge. Here are some examples, as listed in Table 9.1:

Sexual History Questions:

Table 9.1 Reflecting on Meaning Associated with Sexual Experience

What do you remember?	What meaning did you make of that?
What was it like the first time you saw another person naked or saw their genitals?	Was there a sense of interest, embarrassment, confusion? What messages influenced this reaction?
When was the first time you touched yourself in a way that was pleasurable?	Was someone else aware of this? How did their reaction influence the meaning you made of this?

(Continued)

Table 9.1 (Continued)

When was the first time you experienced sexual interest in another person?	Did you know what to do about these feelings? Did you have anyone to ask? How did advice/support, or lack thereof, influence the meaning of the situation?
Did you feel prepared the first time you touched or were touched by someone in a sexual way?	How did knowing/not knowing what to expect influence your experience? What thoughts did you leave with about yourself?

Table offers a column on left that reads sexual health questions based on events that the individual may have experienced, and the column on the right offers question to help the individual reflect on the meaning derived from these experiences

Reflecting on What the Client Wants

In Chapter 5 we used the assessment tool, *"tell me about a recent sexual experience either solo or partnered"* to learn about norms, beliefs, and values. This same question can also be used to help clients reflect on how they evaluate the outcome of their sexual experience. Another helpful question to use alongside this is, *"what did you want to get out of this recent experience?"* For many of our clients, what they wanted may not be clear and often if it is known, it was not achieved. An ideal future template would be for clients to know what they want to achieve and to be able to meet that need or want.

When we are young, we are often told that sex is an expression of love or for making babies. In our peer groups, we often learn that sex is for proving commitment, establishing trust, keeping someone, establishing the relationship or moving it further. For some of our clients, they are caught in between messages they may no longer believe but still influence their values. For many of our clients they have not found the opportunity to reflect on the messages and evaluate what they believe to be true. Enter the clinician, the person to provide this space. Remember the connection to the larger mental/ emotional health realm. What someone does with their body and how they feel about themselves has an enormous impact on functioning and well-being.

Intent, Value Alignment and Outcome

What we expect out of intimacy has countless possibilities. As clinicians we are not seeking a right/wrong answer, rather an alignment of values/beliefs/ desires and an outcome of being able to attain. Some brief examples:

Nina, 25 cisgender, pansexual woman states, "I often pretend for my partner that I am into the romance and the connection but actually, I just get excited lately to try new things out and see what is possible for my body. If I don't get them to orgasm and I don't orgasm but I try something new, I got what I came for."

Dylan, 30, cisgender, gay man states, "I really want to feel connected. Even if it is a hook-up, a brief thing. . . I want to hold him and smell him and just have that connection. Usually, the other person gets off and I don't and I'm totally good with that. . . as long as I get the connection."

As we assist our clients in evaluating their intents/desire/reasons and the outcome, it may become clear that what they want to experience is not often the outcome. There are endless reasons individuals are engaged in sexual experiences that do not meet their needs/expectations. Common reasons include:

Belief that others' sexual needs are more important than one's own

Fear/shame around own sexual desires/needs

Difficulty communicating sexual desires/needs

Lack of information about sexual possibilities (different styles, positions, etc.)

Fear of rejection if desires/needs communicated

Feeling undeserving of pleasure

Feeling uncomfortable expressing pleasure

Needing predictability in sexual experiences

We can become curious about this with clients and also gather some more information to challenge this.

Changing Patterns

Using the guided questions previously discussed, we develop an understanding of what the client wants to experience (sexual values) and the common outcome. We can weave aspects of Strategic Therapy and exposure ladders from Cognitive Behavioral Therapy. In Strategic Therapy we identify and change structural interaction patterns. Applied to sexuality we identify the common pattern and offer suggestions for a different approach. Keep in mind, the change to the pattern is generally difficult, sometimes scary. This is where the exposure ladder concept is helpful. Focus on small changes that offer something different that the client can feel successful at trying. So, the key is trying something different to interrupt a pattern and make that change manageable and small enough.

Here is a step-by-step process:

Step 1: Through guided questions (see previous intervention) client identified a disconnect from desired outcome of sexual experience and actual outcome that is common. Notice this with client.

Step 2: Ask permission to work with client to gather some data.

Step 3: Do Something Different: Focus on desired outcome with client. Consider a new way of exploring intimacy. Like strategic therapy, we aren't trying to identify the ideal outcome, rather simply change the pattern "do something different." Brainstorm a different behavior to change the pattern.

Step 4: Be specific and walk through this new approach. Help the client think through how they will communicate this new way with a partner and consider what feelings may come up for them.

Step 5: Process outcome with client when they report new data (they completed new sexual scenario). If client achieved outcome, meaning their goal/desire aligns with the outcome of their sexual experience, we can help them name what they did to make this possible and how they will advocate for that in future experiences. If the outcome did not align, we may review the situation and make minor changes to help the client approach this again.

Here is a brief example:

Step 1: Kayla reveals that she would like a relationship and to have a sexual experience that was not rushed and shared communication and emotion. She is currently finding partners via dating apps and repeatedly left sad and lonely after hookups.

Step 2: Kayla and therapist agree she will continue her current strategy and gather some data by making some small changes

Step 3: Before determining if a meeting will occur, Kayla agrees that she will ask the potential sexual partner if he is interested in talking for a while over a walk or coffee or drink. She also would like to learn what he would like to do and share what she would like to do sexually, before they begin sexual contact

Step 4: Kayla comes in the next week with data gathered from four hook ups. She used the new tool and noticed it was exciting and empowering to talk about what she wanted. She realized that even though the partners wanted something very different (and one person didn't seem to listen to what she wanted at all), she still went ahead with the sexual experience. As we process this, she realizes she feels obligated at that point to move forward and thinks that this may have led to her misalignment with these partners and again sad and lonely feeling afterward.

Kayla decides in the following week she is going to have the conversation with the potential partner before meeting in person. She would like to increase challenge (exposure ladder, rung 2) by stopping the interaction if their desires for sexual experience do not align.

As you can see from this example, this intervention can help the client gradually change toward behavior that aligns with their sexual value. The processing in Stage 4 is crucial to validating what is difficult and encouraging efforts to modify behavior. Rather than Kayla ending hook ups, the exposure ladder activity helped her specifically challenge her ability to represent her needs and advocate for her sexual pleasure. It also allowed her to take this challenge on at a pace that was not overwhelming and could help her gain confidence with intervals of processing and support.

Listening to the Body and Understanding the Messages

Case Example

LaTonya was a 30-year-old cisgender, heterosexual woman who entered therapy to work on anxiety and relationship difficulties. Early into therapy she identified common experiences of pain when attempting any sexual experience that included penetration. She expressed frustration about how unpredictable her body was. During her biopsychosocial she had not identified any history of major trauma, sexual or otherwise. Using the assessment skill, "tell me about a recent experience," LaTonya shares that she initiated intimacy with her partner after a great movie and cuddle last Saturday. She felt excited to have sex. There was foreplay in the form of kissing and massaging. They both undressed and there was some oral sex and digital sex ("fingering"). She felt excited, eager . . . and then . . . "when he started to go inside me [with his penis] my body just shut down

. . . like he hit a speed bump and he couldn't move deeper." As LaTonya discussed this experience, I was so interested in the term speed bump. She said she just sensed that her body was blocking, slowing down, stopping what was happening. I wondered aloud, "what if you were to listen to the message your body is giving as something informative or helpful instead of frustrating? Speed bumps serve a purpose of slowing us down for some reason of safety. Maybe your body is speaking something your words cannot say at the moment." LaTonya was quiet and thoughtful. She liked the idea of viewing her body as helping her instead of getting in her way. She used this information in the following week and came back with a lot of insight. When she and her partner "hit the speed bump" in a recent experience she just held him and whispered, "let's just pause and stay still for a moment." She was surprised to begin crying and feeling enormous relief. After a few moments they resumed penetration and "the speed bump was gone." As we processed the information, I asked LaTonya what she believed had been different. She reflected that she had always held her body to high expectations, often based on others or the larger society. She offered many examples, running, and pushing her pace and duration, losing weight, even using tampons when they felt uncomfortable in order to fit in with the other girls in gym class. She noted that she rarely thought about her body as a friend or a messenger and often forced it to go beyond its comfort. The idea that her body was informative was a game changer and it had made a huge difference. What was it saying, "slow down and make sure you are comfortable and safe."

Pain, Decrease Erection, Decrease Lubrication – What Is the Body Saying

Pain, discomfort or even a change in how the body is experiencing sensation, should be interpreted as the body's request for attention. Sometimes simply pausing and noticing the sensation can be a 'fix' within itself, like LaTonya's story. We can guide clients to consider short-term and long-term responses to body messages.

Short-term responses to discomfort, pain or change in functioning:

- Pause.
- Consider Context: We are often unaware of all the messages that our bodies are aware of. All of our senses gather information about comfort, excitement, safety in each moment of the day. During sexual excitement

those sensory messages are even more intense. A background noise from a television, a pet entering the room, or even the feeling of something scratchy like stubble could influence pleasure responses. Paying closer attention to the messages in the environment can provide helpful information.

- Make a change: Making a change to context or sensory experience is useful. This might be a change to position, type or degree of touch. This could also be a negotiation with a partner to focus on a different activity or check-in regarding consent and reassurance. Small accommodations such as locking a door, turning down the volume of music, lighting a candle or hydrating are all good to consider.

Long-Term Responses to Discomfort, Pain or Change in Functioning

When desire decreases repeatedly or discomfort or pain occurs in multiple experiences, we should recommend medical intervention to ensure there is not something occurring biologically causing the discomfort or pain. Evaluating when the pain became relevant is important. Stress, fatigue, and health problems often influence sexual pleasure. It is surprising the expectations that many people hold of their bodies to function perfectly without much self-care. Changes to life management and self-care can have a strong correlation to improved sexual pleasure (Rancourt et al., 2015).

Trauma and Disconnection

Pain and discomfort are sometimes difficult for individuals with a trauma history to detect. They may also be hyper-aware of sensations or the possibility of discomfort/pain. Sometimes chronic pain or health problems may be related to an individual not being able to receive the messages of discomfort and change behavior. If there is a history of trauma, especially sexual trauma, asking about awareness of sensations and responses to sensations is very useful. Encouraging the practice of slowing down, listening to the body and trusting the messages of the body is empowering for survivors. As discussed in the *Changing Patterns* intervention, approaching slowly is very important. Disconnecting from the body's messages is often a form of coping, related to trauma. Hearing the messages and feeling the body can be overwhelming. Making incremental change is important.

Consent

Consent is often misunderstood as a one-time, verbal expression of permission. Humans express consent through body messaging, what we say and sometimes what we don't say. We have a responsibility to one another to evaluate many signals, throughout our interactions, to understand consent. Consent, defined by Planned Parenthood:

Freely given

Reversable

Informed

Enthusiastic

Specific

Our culture does very little to respect or teach consent for children. Consider when I child is meeting a new person or a relative, they haven't seen me in a long time. Adults often read shyness as rudeness. Often, they don't ask the child if they would like to give a hug or a fist-bump, rather they demand it, "give your Aunt Kara a hug." Living a healthy and safe life can often mean that we need to learn consent from the very beginning in adulthood. There are wonderful opportunities to help clients practice consent as they navigate therapy services. Giving choices such as, "do you feel safe and comfortable if I close the door of the office for privacy?" Or "when completing the release of information consider what information you would like me to have access to and for how long." Or "does it feel safe to continue talking about this topic?" When there is a discrepancy in the verbal message, tone of voice or body language, we can notice and inquire about this, hopefully increasing the client's awareness about their consent-giving process (Kubota & Nakazawa, 2022).

Sexual interactions are one of the most difficult areas to practice consent. We should help clients practice consent in other domains of functioning and different types of relationships. We can also help them evaluate how they are interpreting consent from others. Some simple activities or "homework" ideas include:

Choose two opportunities to say no to something without explanation. Notice what it feels like in the moment.

Plan an event at work or with a friend and provide details about what you are willing and able to do ahead of time.

Engage in a shared activity with a friend or family member. Pause somewhere in the middle of the activity and check-in to see how they are doing and if they are still wanting to continue on with the activity.

Keep a list of things you agreed to do in the week. Review the list at the end of the week and evaluate what you actually did not want to do or feel comfortable doing. Evaluate why that happened.

In a sexual interaction with someone new it is important to be detailed before initiating physical contact what is agreed to and what is not. Solid start and stop information is extremely helpful. As people may become more familiar with one another, gestures, sounds, and facial expressions may offer additional insight and can be relied on related to consent and boundary setting as well as verbal information.

Sexual experiences have enormous potential to provide pleasure, personal growth, and connection. Most adults did not have access to quality sex education that offered information about sexual pleasure. Most adults are highly influenced by socio-cultural messages and family or religious values that may not align with their current beliefs or lifestyle. For many people sexual performance has little to do with the experience of pleasure. Individuals that have well-understood sexual scripts that align with their own values and desires are safer, healthier, and more confident human beings.

Questions for Reflection and Discussion

Consider a recent experience of discomfort, pain or another type of somatic sensation. Using the tools discussed in this chapter, try to consider the message this feeling may have been trying to share. How might this interpretation change how you responded to your body or the situation?

Are there sexual scripts you have experienced or been exposed to that do not feel healthy? Where did you learn them?

Helping Create a New Normal 10
Addiction, Substance Use, and Sex

Introduction

Throughout history, most cultures have referenced the use of substances related to engagement in sexual intimacy. It is viewed as a relaxant, an aphrodisiac, an inhibitor. For many substances this is in fact true in terms of the subjective experience of desire, and some initial biological processes related to sex. The short-term sense of improvement in the sexual experience often lays the groundwork for addiction or the complicated relationship of substance use and sexual behavior.

Substances and Biological Functioning

Substances that are used recreationally, or, by some, to cope, numb, medicate, generally affect the desire or arousal states of the sexual response cycle.

Alcohol initially increases subjective arousal and in higher amounts, over time, decreases arousal. Common sexual difficulties include, decreased vaginal lubrication, dyspareunia, difficulty or lack of orgasm, erectile difficulty and delayed or inability to ejaculate.

Cannabis increases subjective feelings of pleasure. Chronic use is associated with a decrease in testosterone that may lead to decreased feelings of desire and erection difficulties.

Nicotine use, over time, is associated with erectile difficulties both in obtaining and maintaining erection, decreased vaginal lubrication, and delayed orgasm.

DOI: 10.4324/9781003166382-11

Amphetamines are associated with significant problems related to sexual functioning. The reputation of increased sexual behavior associated with the drug is due to the delay in erection paired with increased desire. In early use, this is often expressed as enjoyable and described as "lasting longer." With prolonged use of the drug increased desire may remain and is paired with erectile difficulty, delayed ejaculation, and anorgasmia.

Cocaine initially induces sexual arousal and increases the quality of the erection. Prolonged use causes erectile difficulty, delayed ejaculation, decreased desire, and delayed orgasm.

Opioids initially cause delayed ejaculation and often decreases pain associated with vaginismus. Prolonged use causes decreased desire and erectile dysfunction.

MDMA initially improves the desire, arousal, and orgasm stages of the sexual experience. The drugs amplification of sensation can lead to an intensity of sexual pleasure when using the drug. For this reason, MDMA is sometimes referred to as "the love drug." Chronic use is associated with erectile dysfunction and delayed orgasm. (Ghadigaonkar & Murthy, 2019)

The impossible standards of sex sold to us in pop-culture can actually be achieved with substances. Harder, longer, ready, relaxed, and exciting are standards that are not realistic but without normalization and education, many people hold themselves to these standards. Without the drugs, the sexual pleasure once experienced will no longer exist.

When many young people are experiencing their first sexual interactions they are also experimenting with substances. For some, especially those that are defined as having substance use disorders, their defining relationships with sex correspond with initial substance use.

The Complicated Relationship of Substances and Sex

As social workers we may engage with clients that are addressing substance use disorder with harm reduction approaches. Other clients may address substance use with abstinence. Many of the clients we encounter will be resistant to treatment and express uncertainty related to the need to change behavior. With all stages of treatment and treatment approaches it is imperative to address sexuality and sexual decision-making as part of each client's substance use treatment. The failure to do so can result in increased harm related to high-risk sexual behavior. Increased risk of relapse is also associated with unaddressed sexual difficulty and concerns during substance disorder treatment interventions (Ghosh et al., 2022).

High-Risk Sexual Behaviors Associated With Substance Use Include

Failure to use protection (condoms, dental dams, PREP, Plan B, other contraception)

Lack of consent due to mind-altering effect of substance

Sex with strangers

Sex in unsafe spaces

Harm to body due to decreased sensation in body during sexual acts

Sexual Difficulties Experienced in Recovery

Increased anxiety

Lack of confidence

Biological consequences of substance

Uncertainty of sexual likes/dislikes

Difficulties feeling desire

Difficulties with sexual expression

Treatment Approaches

Treatment Uncertainty

It is common for clients to disclose a relationship between substance use and sexual behavior. There may be a different presenting concern that causes clients to initiate treatment. Clients may have some uncertainty regarding changing the behavior. Risk may not be heightened during this phase. There may be limited negative consequences for sex and substance use. Useful treatment approaches when motivation is uncertain:

Motivational Interviewing (MI): When clients are in the pre-contemplation or contemplation stage, they benefit a great deal from the opportunity to discuss their thought process. Unlike the direct challenging of some substance use disorder treatment approaches, MI encourages empathy and pacing that is set by the clients. Rather than challenging the client, we develop discrepancy between current behavior and desired goals / behaviors. This can be difficult when clients are in an early stage of substance dependence and sexual behavior. In this early stage, sexual functioning may not be inhibited by substances. Issues of poor decision-making, misunderstanding with partners, and regrets are common concerns. Often resistance is subtle and based in the idea that they will use less of the substance and reduce the negative consequences (Miller & Rollnick, 2013).

Psychoeducation: Information regarding the negative effects of substances on the biological functioning can be useful to the client. Normalizing sexual experiences as imperfect, vulnerable human experiences is also a useful form of education. It may help the client feel less reliant on a substance.

TECHNIQUES

- Assess/reflect on how substances were relied on to improve sexual experience
- Explore new ways to create mood and relaxation
  - Suggestions about the environment (smell, lighting, texture / touch)
  - How to prepare / relax one's self (warm shower or bath, favorite music)
  - Emotional foreplay (planning, sexting, pleasure activities such as favorite foods or dance)

Harm Reduction

Many individuals will never select to address substance use disorder with full abstinence. Harm reduction strategizes with client's current challenges and doesn't require abstinence in exchange for services. The conditions surrounding use, not just the use of the substance, is an area of focus. Clients in this stage are more likely to experience additional negative consequences that they may bring to treatment. They may feel more certain that they need the substance in order to experience desire or other outcomes of sex. Understanding the specific consequences, either biological or relational, is important in helping the client. Exploration for more intensive services can be discussed with clients. Considering the context of substance use and sexual experiences is the primary topic (Bigler, 2005).

Safety planning: Understanding the negative experiences that clients are working to avoid can guide the discussion of a safer or healthier experience. Consent, protection for bodies, safe spaces, and safe people in the environment are important elements to consider in the safety plan. Ideally, a written safety plan that can be evaluated and modified is the most useful approach for clients.

TECHNIQUES

Help clients establish Good – Alright – Bad sex and substance scenarios. Often there is a belief that there are more good times than actually exist. This is a good way to reflect on an increase in negative consequences related to developing discrepancy.

Preparing ahead of substance use is important. Having condoms, Pep, PREP, Plan B, as well as safe words and gestures negotiated with sex partners decreases risk behaviors.

It may be helpful to help the client identify a support person that has permission to intervene in situations that are problematic.

In-Patient or Out-Patient Treatment Program (Abstinence)

Clients that are in a program to detox and recover from a substance will need to establish new ways to approach every domain of functioning. Historically, treatment approaches have failed to address sexuality. There is an increased risk of relapse without therapy focused on sexual needs in recovery. Learning to be sexual without a substance is a completely different, and for some, brand new experience. Feelings of disconnection and failure can often follow individuals as they attempt to initiate personal or shared sexual experiences without substances. Sexuality can be a lifeline for experiencing pleasure, connection, and release for individuals who may have formerly relied on substances for these purposes. Without our help, sexuality can feel scary and out-of-reach when sobriety is the new normal. It is crucial to address this topic directly in recovery (Kumsar, 2016).

> **Grief/Loss**: Individuals may need to mourn the way their body has changed. Often the point of initial substance use is associated with the highest level of sexual pleasure. This is never maintained over the course of use. The emotional and physical consequences related to chronic use and sexual functioning are well-documented. Biological improvements in sexual functioning occur for most individuals when substance use is ended. For some individuals these changes may take six weeks or sometimes six to eight months, depending on course of substance use. Grieving the loss of heightened sexual desire and pleasure is important to acknowledge. The loss of sexual confidence is also common. These losses can lead to isolation.
>
> **Regrets**: Poor decision-making may have resulted in sexual harm. Self-blame is common. Recognition of the effect on emotional and physical health occurs over the course of recovery.
>
> **Sex Education**: Many individuals have little experience being sexual without substances. Basic sex education about how bodies work related to arousal and orgasm is necessary. Important topics include caring for body, consent, and negotiating sexual behavior with partners, healthy expectations for sexual experiences.

Techniques

- Discuss concerns about what may happen sexually/relationally without substances and help client explore new ways to respond.
- Allow for a new experience of knowing one's self. If an individual began their sexual experiences while using substances, they need to begin a practice of learning and exploring. Give permission for nervousness and excitement of learning sexually. See Chapter 11 for specific techniques for self-exploration

"Sex Addiction"

Sex addiction has become an increasingly used term in the last decade. It is generally used by clients or their partners to describe sexual behavior that is either risky, outside the character of the individual or highly repetitive in a way that is causing harm. The term "sex addiction" was initially discussed by Patrick Carnes in the 2001 book, *Out of the Shadows*. Some relief was found in individuals able to identify themselves as having a problem versus the belief they were inherently bad or harmful people. Many mental health professionals have found problem with the sex addiction term and the treatment approach it recommends (Carnes, 2001).

"Sex addiction" is considered an illness and the treatment prescribed is similar to the 12-step-approach that requires recognizing one's self as powerless over the behaviors. Models that reflect the sex addiction approach often pathologize certain types of sex as problematic, resulting in some cases, as heteronormative and kink-shaming. Often approaches require completely abstaining from sexual behavior for some part of the treatment process.

An alternative approach considers the behaviors that feel out of control of the individual to be a sexual health problem. Key to this treatment perspective is the individual's definition of sexual health that informs their motivation for change. Rather than abstinence or condemning any type of sex, developing an understanding of underlying causes for the out-of-control behavior is pursued. The development of a sexual health plan for the individual is also standard to treatment. This approach for the problem labeled by Doug Braun-Harvey and Michael Vigorito as Out of Control Sexual Behavior, is considered by many as sex positive, empowering, and trauma-informed (Braun-Harvey, 2016).

Client Presentations

Sexual behavior that can be described as out of control often lacks pleasure, interferes with functioning, and serves to cope or avoid. Here is some guidance in Table 10.1 on assessment with a client:

We are working to assess if it feels like a problem to the client versus them believing something about the type of sexual behavior is problematic. Viewing pornography, going to strip clubs, masturbating, anal sex, might be viewed by some as "deviant." We are listening not for a type of sexual behavior but the way that it is pursued or completed that is largely unpleasurable, causing difficulty in domains of functioning, possibly causing distress and interfering with other responsibilities. (Braun-Harvey & Vigorito, 2016)

Table 10.1 Assessment for concepts of OCSB

Concepts	What to ask
Sexual behavior that is not enjoyable but often pursued	What do you enjoy about "x?" Or What enjoyment do you get from "x?"
Sexual behavior that interferes with functioning	When you are taking part in "x" behavior, are you still able to take care of work and other responsibilities?
Sexual behavior that serves to avoid or cope with feelings	What sort of feelings, other than desire, cause you to pursue "x" behavior?
Sexual behavior that becomes more excessive or time-consuming	Do you spend more time doing "x" than when you first started doing it?

This table lists concepts of OCSB in the form of specific problems of behavior in the left-hand column. The right-hand column provides questions to ask to assess these behaviors.

Case Study

Martin was in out-patient therapy related to a persistent sad mood and limited motivation. He described his wife as critical and seldom happy with him as a husband or person. He felt overwhelmed with daily responsibilities because he rarely had the energy for his full-time job as an accountant, raising two teenagers, and taking care of the household with his wife. He shared early on that his wife was disappointed that they didn't have sex a lot. He shared that he didn't feel close to her because she was very critical. He completed an Adverse Childhood Experiences (ACE) inventory and had a low score. His interaction within the collaborative, therapeutic relationship demonstrated attributes of a secure attachment. His description of his relationship with his children also described qualities of an individual with a secure attachment (Burke-Harris, 2018).

SW: Martin, it is great to see you again. Thank you for completing the ACE Inventory. It helps me to understand your childhood history because it influences how we function in our relationship with ourselves and in our relationships with others. Your score was low, generally meaning that there were low incidences of adversity or developmental trauma in your childhood.

Martin: I do feel like that's accurate. My parents were both patient people and generally really calm. My wife and I were lucky to have good childhoods and that has helped us agree on a lot in raising our children. We have good relationships with our kids. I'm grateful for that.

SW: You've mentioned that there is some stress in your relationship with your wife. It sounds like that is not related to issues of parenting.

Martin: Nope, we agree on that stuff. She just seems pretty critical of how I interact with her. She often states that she doesn't feel attractive and I don't give her enough attention. I feel pretty confused about what she wants.

SW: Do you feel confused in other relationships? Confused about what people expect or need from you?

Martin: Not really. At work, with my kids, even meeting with you. . . I feel pretty good at communicating. I feel like I make good connections with people.

SW: I can imagine that. It feels like we have created an honest, trusting therapeutic relationship in a short time.

After four weeks of therapy sessions Martin came in especially irritable. He said that his wife said he was a sex addict and told him to "get honest" in therapy. I asked him to tell me more. He shared that he sometimes watched pornography, once or twice a week, in the evenings before bed. They used to watch pornography together as a form of foreplay, but she had lost interest a few years ago. His wife never cared about his viewing habits until she realized that some of his pornography sometimes involved men or multiple people having sex.

I asked Martin some of the questions (identified in this section) related to assessing behavior:

SW: Martin, I'm wondering if you can describe specifically what you enjoy about pornography?

Martin: It is exciting to fantasize about something very different than the sex I have with my wife. Sometimes I watch pornography about threesomes or men having sex with men. I tried to explain to my wife that it is just fantasy, not actually what I want in real life.

SW: It sounds like you feel comfortable with the pornography you watch. You don't have an interest in exploring these types of sexual expression in your own life?

Martin: No, I don't. I used to really enjoy intimacy with my wife. The last few years I have felt really criticized by her and that has actually caused some distance between us.

SW: When you are taking part in watching pornography, are you still able to take care of work and other responsibilities?

Martin: I only porn a couple times a week because most evenings I watch sports with my kids, mow the lawn or watch a movie with my wife.

SW: What sort of feelings, other than desire, cause you to pursue pornography?

Martin: Sometimes curiosity. When I am feeling down or irritable I notice I am less interested in sex or pornography.

SW: Do you spend more time watching pornography now than you did when you first started watching pornography?

Martin: [Took a moment to consider the question.] I think there might have been a slight increase in viewing pornography when I started watching it on my own. In the last two years, the amount of time has not increased. When there is something else in my week, I am fine going without watching it.

SW: From the information you are sharing it sounds like you do not feel concerned about pornography being a barrier or intrusive in your life.

Martin: I think my wife is uncomfortable with the type of pornography I am watching. I wish she understood it is just fantasy, not what I want in my own sexual life. I don't think this is a problem for me, it is more a problem for her.

SW: That may be true. The concept that pornography and erotica depict a fantasy or escape from reality is sometimes misunderstood. Partners sometimes interpret content of pornography as what is preferred in real life and become insulted or concerned. We can't know exactly how your wife is feeling about this but we have come to some clarification about how you feel about your use of pornography. This is really helpful and insightful.

It did seem that there was conflict and misunderstanding in the couple dynamic between Martin and his wife. The exploration in therapy, guided by the assessment questions, allowed me to identify that the behavior Martin's wife had identified as "addictive" or problematic was not out of control for Martin. He watched pornography as an enjoyable activity when he was feeling good versus a behavior that was used to cope, distract or avoid difficult emotions. His behavior had not increased in a way that was interfering with functioning or keeping him from responsibilities in a domain of functioning.

There was other information that was helpful to understand related to Martin's history. Martin did not identify a history of trauma. Histories of abuse and unprocessed trauma are very common among individuals that identify out of control sexual behavior. He also had a lot of protective factors such as relationships with his children, consistent employment, healthy habits of exercise, and hobbies. Health and balance among the multiple domains of functioning, is important for sexual health.

Let's compare Martin's case study to Noah's story.

Case Study

Noah entered out-patient therapy to address a recent divorce and managing parenting responsibilities for his two children. He shared that he and his ex-wife had lots of conflict over parenting issues, intimacy, and finance. They had tried couples therapy but weren't able to resolve their differences.

SW: Noah, I would love to get a sense of a usual day or a usual week in your life. It will help me to understand sources of pleasure and relaxation as well as sources of stress.

Noah: Well, I work a hell of a lot of hours on the computer. I work for a tech firm. I usually get up at the last minute possible to get to my computer. I wish I had time to cook. I usually end up eating a bunch of junk food throughout the day. I've started smoking again. I just generally feel like crap.

SW: It sounds like the hours at work make it really hard to do other things that are important to you.

Noah: Right! I would like to spend more time with the kids. Everything feels behind, like the house is a mess and the lawn is overgrown.

SW: I noticed when you completed the log of your time over the course of last week there was "work" listed and then "research" or "computer." Are those extra hours that you are working that you aren't paid for?

Noah: No, not work. I wish. If it were work or anything useful I probably wouldn't be so behind. It is just surfing porn. Sometimes I do that just to check out, relieve stress. In the long run it probably doesn't because it makes me guilty and puts me behind with everything else.

SW: I can see how that might get in the way. Some of the days last week it was three or four hours marked as "research" or "computer." What is the guilt about?

Noah: Well, the things I care about aren't getting attention because I just lose track of time once I start surfing porn.

SW: Is this something that has been happening for a while?

Noah: Oh, even my ex-wife got on me about it. She didn't have a problem with porn but she had a problem with all the time that I lost to it. She said that I didn't know how to stop. She's probably right.

SW: What sort of feelings prompt you to start watching porn?

Noah: It is different than the desire I feel if I am interested in someone. I have a lot of times when I get overwhelmed by feeling not good enough and I think I go to porn and masturbating to get rid of, maybe distract from that feeling.

SW: Do you feel that it actually helps with that?

Noah: Well, I get zoned out for the time I'm doing it. When I finally stop I just feel worse than when I started. Then I am guilty and feel bad about myself because I'm more behind.

Noah had already identified that the amount of time he was spending was interfering with other domains of functioning. He identified that the behavior wasn't enjoyable because it interfered with his life and didn't actually make him feel better. When he eventually stopped watching the pornography, he felt guilt.

As Noah continued in therapy, he revealed a history of physical and sexual abuse in his childhood. The shame he referenced when we were completing assessment questions was rooted in this childhood trauma. The treatment plan required processing this trauma history. Treatment also included helping Noah identify his motivation for healthy sexuality and developing a unique plan to reach his sexual health goals.

Unlike Martin's case, Noah reflects on the use of viewing pornography as an interference with his functioning. He doesn't pursue pornography based on sexual pleasure but rather to numb or distract from negative emotions. In Noah's case, a great deal of the negative emotions were associated with experiences of abuse in his childhood. He had never had the opportunity to process these experiences or begin a healing journey. Sexual behaviors became one of his only ways to cope with the negative and overwhelming feelings.

Treatment Approaches

Trauma-Informed

The mental health professional addresses the problem from a trauma-informed lens. The clinical experience related to individuals with OCSB points to a strong history of trauma, often attachment or developmental injuries that are foundation for the behavior. This is often not within the realm of awareness of the client when they begin seeking treatment.

The behavior is understood as a form of self-soothing. OCSB within its definition is often limited or without pleasure. Sexual experiences are most often pursued without understanding of why, are limited or without pleasure and feel beyond the control of the individual to limit or stop the behavior. The individual lacks multiple coping strategies to manage difficult emotions and needs to both understand this (psychoeducation) and develop these resources in treatment.

Behavior Defined by Client

The problem is not a problem of sex. Often group or 12-step approaches seek to "fix" addictive or out of control sexual behavior through abstinence or limiting the types of sexual behaviors. Helping individuals develop healthy coping mechanisms and a healthy relationship with their sexual needs/desires is imperative to treatment. Developing an understanding of the difference between soothing and pleasure is also key to treatment.

Sexual Health Plan

Helping clients create a balanced life of sexual pleasure and safety requires open dialogue about their own sexual needs, values, and decision-making about sexual choices. The development of a sexual health plan addresses the following areas:

> Consent involves having a willing partner that is capable of joining in a sexual experience that is of an age of consent, and can choose to join in a sexual experience fee of invasive, intrusive or violating methods. Consent occurs in every step of the sexual experience. It creates the opportunity for safety and pleasure consistent with one's own sexual desires.
>
> (Coleman, 2002)

Non-exploitative sexual experiences are free of power and control related to sexual gratification. The partners involved can consent to every experience without threat of losing something or having something negative occur to them based on their decision to/not to participate in the sexual experience.

Honest communication takes place with one's self and partner(s) regarding sexual pleasure and sexual health.

Shared values are the sexual standards and ethics that govern the specific sexual experiences an individual is motivated to take part in. Sexual values influence motivation for sex across the lifespan. Conversation about sexual values is necessary between partners because differences often exist and can be harmful if not openly explored.

Protection from HIV, STI, and unwanted pregnancy is a need for anyone engaged in sexual activity. It includes quality sexual information and education, a plan to utilize contraception and prevent sexually transmitted infection.

Pleasure to explore sexual interests in balance with sexual safety and responsibility is a continuous and changing motivation across the lifespan. Respecting what brings us sexual pleasure and sexual curiosity and how that may be different from others is necessary to uphold safety and health for ourselves, our partners and our communities.

A sexual health plan is unique to each person and should define the six elements of sexual health and consent. It also identifies a routine of self-care and connection that can be followed. In helping individuals develop new ways of coping and soothing on a daily basis it is less likely they will rely on sexual behavior as a form of soothing (Braun-Harvey, 2016).

Noah's Sexual Health Plan:

It is necessary to define healthy sexuality from the client's perspective. This should include the elements: consensual, non-exploitive, protective, shared values, and mutual pleasure.

Noah described healthy sexuality this way:

When dating a new partner he would discuss ahead of time the sexual expression that felt pleasurable and exciting to him and learn this about his partner too. He identified wanting to be sober when making sexual decisions. He identified that he would not pressure a partner or become quiet or withdrawn if there is a limit or a hard no related to sexual behavior. He identified that checking in after a sexual experience about what felt good and maybe where there was uncertainty would help him gain trust with the person and also hold him accountable.

In addition to healthy sexuality, the sexual health plan covers new habits. This includes healthy habits in the individual's lifestyle that supports wellness and good decision-making.

Noah identified several new habits:

- Working out in the morning before starting work
- Cooking meals at the beginning of the week so he could eat better throughout the week
- Communicating with friends on a daily basis

- Having clear boundaries about starting and stopping work
- Having a weekly outing with his kids
- Communicating with the children's mother about coparenting on a routine basis

A sexual health plan should also include replacement behaviors. Clients need help identifying what they will do instead of the behaviors that have led to negative consequences.

Noah identified several replacement behaviors:

- Go for a walk when feeling overwhelmed
- Facetime a friend when feeling "not good enough"
- Read over personal affirmations when negative self-talk is prominent

It is also useful to identify the negative pattern that leads to the out-of-control behavior. Initially clients may think that "it just happens." By exploring a recent event, a pattern can be identified. This pattern includes:

> **Triggers**: the reminders, feelings, events, thoughts that bring about the bad feelings
>
> **Risky situation**: this is something that leads the individual a step closer to the problematic behavior
>
> **Self-talk rationalization**: the phrases the individual tells themselves to justify negative behavior
>
> **Giving up**: the thought and behavior that signals the individual is no longer trying to avoid the negative behavior
>
> **Problematic behavior**: define specifically what this behavior is for the individual
>
> **Consequences**: this may include emotions, legal, relational or physical consequences

Noah identified this pattern:

- Triggers: feeling unhealthy, feeling tired and behind at work, feeling disconnected from friends and family
- Risky situation: staying home alone, returning to computer when he has decided he is done working
- Self-talk rationalization: "I'll just be here for a second. I deserve a break"
- Giving up: Looking at search history on computer

- Problematic behavior: opening porn site
- Consequences: feeling unworthy, feeling guilty, missing out on time with kids, getting behind in all responsibilities

A sexual health plan allows the mental health clinician to identify the healthy lifestyle behaviors that support sexual health. It provides the client autonomy and responsibility to define sexual health for themselves within the guidelines of the principles. Checking in on the sexual health plan, clients may share that they have difficulty keeping to the plan. Using the therapeutic relationship, we can explore with curiosity what is competing with their motivation toward their commitment. Sometimes we may note ambivalence and encourage the client to consider what feels manageable or what they might be willing to do, if not the entire goal. For example, Noah may not be willing to commit to working out in the morning, but he is willing to get up on time and do a few stretches before starting his day.

The information provided in this chapter will help social workers explore sexual choices and decision-making that may be confusing or overwhelming for clients. The assessment information discussed in this chapter will guide conversations that allow clients to define their own sexual motivations and conflicts. Out of control sexual behavior is not about a type of sexual behavior. When sexual behaviors are used to cope with difficult emotions as a form of avoidance and soothing it can often become excessive and inhibit well-being. Specific trauma-informed treatment may be necessary to address an individual's history of abuse and mistreatment. This may include approaches such as Eye Movement Desensitization Reprocessing (EMDR). OCSB can lead to high-risk behavior that puts clients, and possibly others, at significant legal, emotional, and physical risks. A safety plan in addition to a sexual health plan is recommended to establish and regularly evaluate/update with clients. Supervision is crucial when behaviors involve harm to self/others.

Questions for Reflection and Discussion

What emotions exist for professionals surrounding clients on-going struggle or pain in a harm-reduction model of treatment?

What difficulties could exist in individual or couples work if you were to challenge the idea of sex addiction? What language would you use to discuss the difference between sex addiction and OCSB?

Biopsychosocial Treatment Approaches

11

Introduction

Intervention plans are unique to each client. They are shaped by goals and objectives associated with the presenting problems and symptoms identified in assessment. In our changing mental health field and the sex therapy field, treatment approaches are often based in somatic experiences. Treatment approaches that touch on the emotional, intellectual, creative, spiritual, and relational yield the greatest growth for clients.

Developing an Intervention Plan:

PLISSIT is a model developed by psychologist Jack Anon to help determine the differing level of intervention an individual may need. The model works to ensure that practitioners are intervening at the most basic level first. This model encourages the practitioner to be guided prominently by the client's comfort level and interest in engaging in specific interventions. In terms of social work, the PLISSIT model is broadly comparable to the concept of resourcing and case management versus in-patient or intensive-outpatient therapy. In most cases we attempt to intervene to address a presenting problem in the least invasive manner possible. The PLISSIT Model follows this framework:

P = Permission

LI = Limited Information

SS = Specific Suggestions

IT = Intensive Therapy

DOI: 10.4324/9781003166382-12

While PLISSIT was introduced in 1976, it was retitled by Sally Davis and Bridget Taylor in 2006 as the EX-PLISSIT model. This new title sought to highlight the importance of the permission phase of the model (Tuncer & Oskay, 2022). Acknowledging the client's ownership in their own voice and sexuality is the cornerstone of the Permission stage. The understanding that giving voice to an experience, naming, and receiving connection, and validation of that experience is important and often healing in and of itself, is also key to the Permission stage (Taylor & Davis, 2007).

We can incorporate the PLISSIT model into any stage of treatment either during the primary assessment or when a specific concern arises during treatment. The use of PLISSIT can often help us determine the source(s) of the presenting symptoms. If the symptom has been lifelong or acquired, generalized or situational, may become apparent during the PLISSIT process. We are both assessing and offering interventions in the PLISSIT model.

The following is an example of the PLISSIT model with a client:

Permission: create the space for the discussion of sexual health, "are there any topics related to sexual health that you would like to discuss?"

During an initial assessment, Andrea shares that she experiences high anxiety in lots of social situations. She mentions that she is eager to have a sexual relationship with her girlfriend but is worried that she will do something wrong. The therapist asks if Andrea would be interested in talking about this topic in more detail. Andrea agrees. The therapist reiterates the importance of Andrea feeling in charge of the content and pace of the conversation. Andrea is reminded that pausing or stopping the discussion about the topic is always her choice.

Limited Information: Responding to the concern with limited information related to the potential source of the problem. This is a form of psychoeducation.

The clinician shares that anxiety related to sexual performance is a common concern. Having a conversation about sexual interests and preferences can often increase insight and relieve concerns. Asking permission to share some of your own sexual values often opens the door to a partner to share their likes/dislikes and nervousness as well.

Specific Suggestions: Andrea shares that she doesn't really know what she likes to do so she feels scared to talk about it. We discuss some books as well as a YouTube channel produced by a sex educator that discusses lots of sexual topics in a fun, approachable manner. Andrea feels excited to take a look at these resources before attempting to talk to her girlfriend.

Intensive Therapy: Sometimes limited information and specific suggestions clearly do not offer resolution. More intensive or involved time and resources will need to be dedicated to the topic. We might respond by saying, "it sounds like this issue is a bit more complicated to resolve all at once. Can we agree to work on this more specifically in a coming session?" In some settings that don't allow for more involved therapy, a referral for therapy would be provided at this time.

For Andrea, intensive therapy for this topic is not required.

If we return to the case study of Janice from Chapter 5, we can image that the PLISSIT model would result in a referral for or need for more intensive therapy. Remember that Janice shared that there was little sexual pleasure in her life. She had sex with her husband once a week because she felt she needed to do this, she didn't feel desire to do this. She felt resentful and often used alcohol to numb her feelings in order to have sex. The limited information and specific suggestions of the PLISSIT Model would likely result in discussion of underlying issues that included history of sexual assault, lack of communication in primary relationships. In mental health, as well as the medical profession, we offer the least invasive strategy to address the concern. We also listen closely for underlying issues that may need more intensive care.

When underlying issues are the cause of sexual difficulties we must understand "the thread" that weaves together relational, mental, sexual, and emotional challenges. History of trauma, health difficulties and pain disorders, attachment injuries, desire difficulties, body image issues are some of the major themes we identify. When selecting appropriate interventions, we must consider the type of issue we are attempting to address.

Empowerment Interventions

These interventions increase insight related to the body. They offer the opportunity to practice skills of consent and communication. They can be experienced as empowering as well as a type of exposure therapy because they require trying out a new form of communication about vulnerable topics. These could be useful for individuals with a history of sexual, physical or emotional abuse. Individuals that have previously been or are currently diagnosed with gender dysphoria, body dysmorphia or an eating disorder may also benefit from these interventions. This can be especially powerful for gender non-binary and transgender clients to experience the power of naming and introducing their body with the language that fits. Individuals or couples that are working to improve communication and practices of consent may also benefit.

Naming Exercise

The Naming Exercise asks the client to introduce each part of their body with the name they use for it. After naming the body part they can express how they feel about this part of their body and any history about this body part. For example:

> "This is my forehead. My partner calls it my worry mat because of all the wrinkles that appear when I'm deep in thought. I'm actually embarrassed about my worry mat as I get older because it makes me appear older."

Another example is, "this is my front hole (in reference to a vagina). I don't like it. It has lots of bad memories and now it reminds me of times I've been viewed as a girl and that is upsetting."

The clinician serves as a witness in the exercise. Process questions are useful.

> How does it feel to name that part of you?
>
> Has the relationship with this part of your body changed over time?
>
> What is it like for this part of you to have attention?

Modifications to this intervention include:

> Inviting a partner to serve as witness
>
> Having a couple introduce parts to one another
>
> Placing written text over body parts that feel too hard to name.

Role Play and Sexual Scripts

There are many versions of this intervention.

> **Practicing consent**: An individual or couple can discuss a scenario that has occurred or a scenario they would like to occur. They can practice introducing what they want, asking questions, setting limits. The clinician may play a role as other partner, or simply pause and give feedback, or make suggestions.

Revisiting a dialogue: We could use this method with an individual or couple to address a difficulty in communication of sexual needs. Begin by asking the client to describe what they are hoping for from the sexual experience. Ask them to imagine they are speaking to their partner and practice the interaction. The clinician can note areas that are unclear or would benefit from some type of revision. When done with a couple, it is useful to pause and help the other partner to ask clarifying questions or share their own wants or feelings.

We can also use this intervention to explore a scenario that is shameful, traumatic or regretted. The client can begin by recalling what was said and what did occur. Recalling and remembering is healing in itself when there is trauma, shame or grief. The scenario is then recalled a second time. This time the client inserts what they wanted to say or do but felt unable. Processing the experience by exploring:

How did it feel different to say what you wanted or needed to say?

How did it feel in your body the first time, the second time?

Can you remember what stood in your way of being able to say these things at the time?

Mirror Activity

This may be used when changes occur to the body from illness, injury or accident have occurred. It may also be useful for body shame related to trauma or negative view of the body.

The activity, done all at once, should only be approached by a client that expresses feeling enthusiastic and will likely not be overwhelmed with the experience. Otherwise, consider offering the activity in steps.

Establish a place of privacy. Stand in front of a mirror naked. If naked is too overwhelming the client can consider wearing a top and underwear or something similar. Ask the client to slowly scan the body from top to bottom. They may want to begin facing front and then turn to side to notice their body from different perspectives. You can ask them to record feelings or thoughts they notice about different parts of their body. When processing this material in the future session this written recording of this experience can be used to consider:

How did this feeling about this part of you develop?

Are there things about this part of your body you can be grateful or appreciative for?

How would things feel different if you had a positive belief about this part of your body?

How do you imagine others feel about this part of your body? How do you know?

Modifications to this exercise:

For clients that may be overwhelmed by looking at their naked body in entirety, you can suggest they examine parts at a time. Begin with an arm or foot and have them record emotions and thoughts that arise.

If the client needs additional distance, they can take a photograph of the body part and view the photograph.

Clients that experience body dysmorphia or gender dysmorphia may benefit from first, drawing specific body parts the way that they view them in their mind. Then they can compare how the drawing is different from their actual body. Developing discrepancy between the belief and the actual is necessary. The discrepancy can then be discussed.

Repeat the same processing questions already described.

Body Exploration

Individuals that experience injury, illness or some type of change to their body may initially experience loss and limitations related to sexual experience. We can use the interventions in this section to expand the map of the body. The client can learn new ways to experience sexual pleasure that are less impacted by the injury, illness or change.

Individuals that experience low desire and limited sexual scripts can benefit from these interventions to learn more about their body and sexual possibilities.

Individuals that experience any chronic pain and/or genito-pelvic pain disorder can learn to focus on parts of their body that offer sexual pleasure that are not the source of pain or discomfort.

Individuals that have experienced sexual trauma often struggle with pain, decreased desire or heightened triggers or flashbacks related to touch on certain parts of their body. Learning to change the messaging of touch, or even find new ways to be touched, can be very empowering and relieving.

Individuals that are gender non-binary or transgender can use these interventions to discover expansive ways to experience sexual pleasure.

Body Map

Body maps are used to address a diversity of presenting concerns within many modalities of therapy. Mental health professionals may use body maps to identify areas of pain, notice somatic symptoms or address self-harm and eating disorders. The body map was referenced in Chapter 5 as an assessment approach. It is useful to initially use this to gather information and then readdress the body map as an intervention. During the intervention, we are guiding clients to understand the reasoning of the messages they have about their body, learn to communicate about their body map, and also expand their sexual scripts to increase safety and pleasure based on the body map. The steps to these interventions can be modified based on the specific concerns of the client.

If the client created a body map as part of the interactive assessment process, the clinician can revisit the map with the client during treatment. If there was not a map created during assessment:

- Provide an outline of a body on a piece of paper. One outline for the front of the body, one for the back of the body. You can draw this freehand, ask the client to draw it or download a simple body outline from the internet.
- Ask the client to color the outline identifying (green) parts of the body they like to be touched sexually (yellow); maybe areas they are interested in exploring or they're willing to consider; or not sure (red) parts of the body they do not want to be touched.
- Discuss the outlines, front, and back, with the client. Focus on the reasons for green/yellow/red identification and inquiring about narratives related to specifically green or red body parts.
- Ask the client to number the green parts of the body from one (begin here) to ending number as a way to describe their ideal way of being touched sexually.
- Discuss with the client the ways that they like to be touched in each area. This might include rubbing, stroking, pinching, massaging, etc.
- Inquire about the areas of the body that are identified by yellow (maybe). Help the client to be curious about what types of touch might be

interesting to them. Ask the client to imagine a sexual interaction and how they might communicate with a partner about the parts of body that are identified in yellow.

- Ask the client to imagine a sexual interaction that they communicate about the parts of the body labeled red (no zones).

Modifications to the intervention:

When working with couples or inviting a partner into a session, the clinician can create a space to allow the partners to share body maps. Be thoughtful about the process of this interaction. Help the couple consider if they can ask for additional information from one another. Consider what feedback might be helpful before beginning the activity.

Mindful-Touch (based on components of Sensate Focus)

Sensate Focus is a specific sex therapy invention to increase awareness in a mindful and sensory-focused encounter(s). The activity is not designed to be erotic but rather mindful. It helps individuals explore the reactions of their own body and learn about their partner's body. There are several steps to the Sensate Focus intervention originally described by sex researchers, Masters, and Johnson. I would not recommend applying the entirety of the Sensate Focus activity without additional sex therapy training. The following steps offer modification to Sensate Focus that is less involved but allows for exploration of the body. It can serve to expand insight and increase connection between partners (Linschoten et al., 2016).

Key concepts that this intervention will used that are derived from the original Sensate Focus intervention include:

Exploration of sensory experience in touch using temperature, texture, and pressure

Non-demand touching with a focus on gaining insight versus arousal

Mindful Touch intervention is useful for individuals that are seeking to expand knowledge of their own body to improve experiences of desire or arousal. It is sometimes described as mindfulness for touching and in this way can be useful for individuals that experience anxiety, pain or past trauma related to the body or sexual experiences. The purposes are quite expansive. Detailed instructions are provided by the clinician. The intervention is completed on the client's own schedule and then processed in future interaction with the clinician.

- Begin with an introduction of purpose with the client. It is best described as a mindfulness activity to increase awareness about touch. Determine if the client will be exploring this individually or with a partner based on the current personal/relational context of the client. Some clients may want to approach it on their own and then introduce a partner at a future time. The original Sensate Focus is only done in partnership.

- Ask the client to consider a space in their home that is peaceful and offers privacy. It can be useful to brainstorm with clients that may have difficulty securing this in their own spaces. Ideas about lighting to increase peacefulness, peaceful music, locking a door or even aromatherapy via a spray or candle are all helpful ideas to create peace in the space.
- Suggest that the client finds 20–30 minutes for each mindful activity.
- Help the client determine if they will complete the mindfulness on their own or with a partner. If a partner is involved ensure that each person understands the purpose and agrees to focusing on mindfulness versus arousal.
- Props that can be helpful might include a heated therapy pillow, ice cubes, lotion, massage oil, hand-held or finger massager.
- The client should lie on their back on the floor or bed. If it is a partnered activity, they should determine who will be the toucher/touched and then switch out after 10 minutes.
- Consider focus areas of the face, neck, shoulders, arms, hands, lower legs, and feet.
- An individual should begin at their forehead, first noticing different types of touch on the forehead and over the nose and lips. This may include gentle strokes with a fingertip and moving to gentle taps on the forehead and cheekbones followed by a deeper pressure. They should notice how these different types of touch are experienced.
- Help them think through interchanging ideas of temperature, texture, pressure with the different props they are able to bring to the activity. Encourage them to be curious without strict rules for the process. Providing a few examples might set the process in motion in their mind. Begin with the ideas for the face and then suggest changing things on their shoulders or legs to include lotion or cold/hot.
- Partners should follow a similar process as described for the individual with a consistent individual first being the toucher and then switching when they arrive at completion of the body. Hand-riding can be suggested so that the individual receiving touch can guide the touching by placing their hand on top of the person touching. This can help them remain mindful and non-verbal while still providing some information about how they are receiving the touch.
- Journaling after the mindfulness activity can offer insights that can be discussed in a future session.

- It is terrific to check in about how the activity influenced calmness and relaxation related to touch. Identifying if there is new information about parts of the body or types of touch may help the client to expand how they explore desire/arousal in the future.

Modifications

Sex therapists use many modifications of this intervention to increase insight. Sensate Focus moves into genital and breast touching, exploring this activity naked and working toward penetrative experiences. The intervention of mindful touch does not intend to progress in those directions.

Focusing more on planning the props used would be an important element for an individual who has little insight into their body or pleasure. Allowing them space to brainstorm and be curious can be highlighted as part of the intervention.

Focusing on moving to different parts of the body and changing the focus in one's mind is an area of the intervention that should be highlighted for individuals that are fixated on problems with arousal or performance of their body.

Redirecting

Most individuals have a tendency to over-focus on a sexual difficulty. The difficulty may be pain or perhaps difficulty maintaining an erection. The more the difficulty is thought about, the larger it becomes. One of the major reasons that sex therapy focuses on expanding the map of sexual pleasure to the entire body, is to help individuals fixate less on "the parts that aren't working." We don't want to introduce the intervention of redirection in the case of clients avoiding a larger problem related to intimacy. With redirection we are very simply walking clients through moving their focus. It is similar to a thought replacement used in Cognitive Behavioral Therapy for any number of presenting concerns.

- Notice a fixation held by the client. This may be pain in sexual experience, erection, breast size, etc.
- Ask the client how this problem interferes with them having sexual pleasure.
- Provide psychoeducation that may include catastrophic thinking from CBT or WISE Mind from DBT.

- WISE Mind: observe thoughts and feelings and describe them without judgement.
- Catastrophic Thinking: What is the concern? How likely is it to happen? What is the worst part of it if it does occur? (Follette et al., 2014)
- Ask the client to consider their body map (if they have completed one) or Mindful Touch exercise and identify an alternative area or behavior that brings pleasure.
- Ask them to complete a guided visualization:
- Picture yourself enjoying an intimate experience with –
- Notice that you become aware of – (insert specific problem).
- Let yourself name that problem in your head and simply observe that it is happening
- Redirect your attention to your other body part/behavior.
- Notice the way that you will also give direction to your partner to change the focus.
- Imagine enjoying this new experience.

Once the client is able to master this visualization, they may want to add the step of imagining going back to the problem focus and visualizing it improved

The next step in this intervention is the client completing this experience in reality. Pace this with readiness and continue using the visualization until they feel a sense of confidence.

Naming Pain

The belief that pain provides a message can often help individuals change their belief or relationship to pain. When we are working to make pain stop, it can sometimes create a cycle of fear and pain and anxiety. Some simple steps can guide clients to engage with pain in a more useful manner.

- Think about where the pain occurs and when it occurs. Ask the client to image that the pain is offering a message.
- Consider naming the pain. Give it a name that is associated with the message. Examples might include, slow down, rest, watch out.
- Complete a brief visualization.
- Ask the client to imagine the experience of pain in their body at this moment.
- Send a few deep breaths to the pain.
- Name it in your mind and observe.

Practicing naming pain in combination with redirecting intervention can be extremely useful for individuals experiencing chronic pain or sexual pain.

Expanding the Script

Many individuals are negatively influenced by the limited and often problematic cultural messaging related to sexuality and intimacy. This results in a fear of behaving outside a perceived "sexual norm." Inviting clients to be curious and allow themselves to own their fantasies may open the door to learning more about their unique sexuality. As clinicians, it is important that we offer normalization of the full expanse of sexual expression. We do not need to speak directly for the client regarding their sexual preferences, but we can generalize suggestions. We might state:

> "Most fantasies allow us to imagine experiences that are very different from our daily lives. Fantasies can offer an escape. They are not necessarily what we actually want for ourselves but rather are an imaginative form of play."
>
> "Lots of people incorporate some form of kink into their sexual repertoire. Kink may be about ways of dress, role play, power or sometimes pain. Certainly, there are many ways to practice kink and you don't have to like them all to consider trying some."

Clients may have repressed parts of their sexual selves and need permission to consider or discuss things they feel interest in. Clinicians can normalize, educate, and then provide resources for additional information.

Useful Modalities

Therapy modalities that align particularly well with sex therapy include Internal Family Systems (IFS) and Eye Movement Desensitization Therapy (EMDR). Additional training is required to establish yourself as trained or certified within these modalities. Particular elements of these modalities allow the sexual domain to be understood as a thread that is woven into the other domains of functioning.

Internal Family Systems, developed by Richard Schwartz, considers the multiplicity of the mind. The parts as protectors and the exiles often intervene when the "Self" is in some way in need of protection. IFS views behaviors often viewed as maladaptive in other modalities as behaviors to be seen as parts trying to help. The sexual difficulties that have been discussed in this book, compulsive behaviors, co-occurring disorders, sexual pain, abuse, and trauma, are an expression of difficulty and also serve as a way of trying to help or protect the "Self." IFS interventions, aimed at understanding and providing compassion for parts, provides a wonderful pathway of integration (Schwartz, 2020).

Eye Movement Desensitization Reprocessing (EMDR), developed by Francine Shapiro, utilizes dual attention stimulus to process distressing experiences to reduce distress and increase positive cognitions of the self. Often negative experiences of the past or negative beliefs about safety, control, and responsibility become expressed by or interwoven in sexual experiences. The use of EMDR to heal presenting problems directly allows integrated memories to surface and be processed. Similar to IFS, increased insight and acceptance generally accompany the process (Shapiro, 2017).

Case Study: Reflecting on Janice

Janice was introduced as a case study in Chapter 5. Janice's story helped to illustrate the case conceptualization and understanding *the thread* of patterns and themes. The assessment process opened the presenting problems of low motivation, lack of pleasure and decreased energy, and revealed themes of lack of support and disconnection, trauma, dissociation, numbing, and health concerns. During the assessment process it becomes clear that there is a *thread* that connects all of these themes together. It is through the interventions that Janice reveals her story to herself and her mental health provider. It is in this story and the processing that she begins to heal.

At the end of the assessment phase Janice experienced an "ah ha" moment connecting the sexual pain she experienced with the shame and disconnect from her own body. She felt disempowered and lacked communication related to sexual feelings. She felt unseen by her mother, her family, her husband. She carried a deep resentment in the relationship with her husband and forcing herself to have sex with her husband reminded her of her sexual trauma.

Beginning with the PLISSIT Model it was quickly revealed that specific suggestions would do little to touch the long-term problems with sex, mood, and relationships that Janice experienced. In the beginning phase of treatment Janice often entered sessions in a rush. She felt disheveled and often complained about how she looked and how poorly her clothes fit. Inquiring about her feelings about her body, it felt appropriate to suggest the naming intervention. "I'm wondering if you would try something?" I inquired. "Would you mind approaching a brief exercise that allows you to give a name, whatever name you choose, to each part of your body." Janice rolled her eyes and sighed. "Sure, I'll give it a shot. I guess just start at the top?" she said pointing to her hair.

She began, "limp, graying hair [pointing at head], headache center [pointing at forehead], food factory [pointing to mouth]." She began to cry, seeming to notice the negative beliefs early in this exercise. "Tits, that's what Dan calls them" [pointing to her breasts and referencing her husband]. It took almost 20 minutes to finish and we never got past her hips.

As we processed the experience, Janice noted that the bad feelings about herself had grown significantly. She described feeling initially scared to have the attention on her body but also, very seen, in a compassionate way through the exercise. She ended by saying, "all this stuff that has happened to me is just playing out on this body of mine." We continued to reflect on the stories associated with the different parts of her body in future sessions.

We modified the mirror exercise. I asked Janice to take a photo of a part of her body she likes and a part that she used to like and no longer likes. She brought in a photo of her hand in the next session. She told me the story of her hands that care for her children and work in the garden. She loved how rough they felt. She said that "the wear and tear was all from things I love to do." She showed me a picture of her cleavage. She remembered that she once felt sexy in high school, but now this part of her just felt "droopy and overused." In processing, Janice imagined that feeling differently about her chest and other body parts would allow her to be confident and out-going like the other moms that she visits with in the neighborhood. She said that she wanted that confidence but it felt out of reach.

Janice's desire to feel differently about her body also revealed the importance of self-care and developing a new relationship with her body. I discussed the Mindful Touch exercise. The hardest part was establishing privacy. This took her more than two weeks. After completing the initial 20 minutes on her own she was very surprised that it was enjoyable. She even noticed that some "sexy thoughts" came up that evening. She said, "it was like some part of me just woke up through that time." Janice noted that she wanted to feel better and learn to do things good for herself.

In thinking about the self-care and good ways of taking care of herself, we also reflected on the harm of having sex when she didn't want it. We used the Revisiting Dialogue exercise to imagine a recent sexual experience. When I asked Janice to revisit specific moments in the interaction and say what she actually wanted to say, a large amount of anger surfaced. Her voice was raised and tears spilled out of her eyes. She yelled, "I just want to tell him, do you even care what I want?. . . or do you just want to do me?" The processing of this exercise took several sessions and the question: What stood in the way of saying what you wanted? lead us back to the beginning, to her initial sexual trauma.

During Janice's treatment we used Internal Family Systems Therapy and Eye Movement Desensitization Reprocessing often. The interventions of Naming, the Mirror Activity, Revisiting Dialogue, were enormously helpful in allowing Janice to discover *the thread* that wove her story. Janice left therapy having processed her trauma. She established terrific boundaries with people in her life. She found pleasure first in her own sexual exploration, and then she was able to establish that with her husband.

The interventions of this chapter are certainly not an exhaustive list. They require that we use the skill of witnessing, noticing, and processing to deliver reflection and process experiences. I hope that you can use the detailed steps to begin this work with your own clients.

The use of the PLISSIT Model provides a framework for educating and approaching sexual difficulties with specific solutions. It is always important to offer additional referrals when a problem is consistent or has a medical component. Chapter 13 provides details on networking and referrals.

Medical Referrals

Gynecologist

Individuals with a vulva/vagina that are experiencing pain in sexual activity should seek care from a gynecologist. When pain is an issue or history of sexual abuse, gynecological exams can be very anxiety-producing. Gynecologists, physician assistants, and nurse practitioners that have an AASECT Sex Counseling Certificate have specific training to address these issues with support and pacing that will aid the client.

Individuals that are sexually active and have not had gynecological services should be encouraged to have an exam. Referrals should be provided when an individual has a new sexual partner for STD testing, HIV testing, and information regarding contraception. Transgender men that have a vagina, uterus or ovaries will require gynecological care and it is important to decipher the doctors in your network that will offer the best support, safety, and advocacy for transgender care (Hogben et al., 2015).

Other common problems that can cause pain in sexual experiences include endometriosis, interstitial cystitis, menopause, and uterine fibroids. Vaginismus and dyspareunia may also be diagnosed or treated in gynecology or pelvic floor physical therapy.

Urology

Individuals that experience problems with blood flow that lead to erectile difficulty should initially see a primary care physician and may be referred to a urologist. Urologists also treat ejaculation problems, injury to the penis, nerve disorders and Peyronie's disease, a painful curvature of the penis due to plaque build-up.

Pelvic Floor Physical Therapy

Pelvic floor physical therapists are physical therapists with a specialization in pelvic floor pain. Urinary dysfunction for individuals with a penis or vagina may be treated by a pelvic floor physical therapist. Sometimes erectile dysfunction is also treated by this specialization. Vaginismus and dyspareunia are commonly treated by pelvic floor physical therapists.

Questions for Reflection and Discussion

When considering readiness and pacing, what might we look for in client expression or behavior before introducing the Mindful Touch exercise?

How would you interpret and address client avoidance of one of these treatment approaches?

Honoring the Diversity of Sexual Expression

12

Introduction

Being aware of the limitations and bias you may bring to the topic of sexuality and intimacy is necessary in order to show up as an authentic mental health practitioner. Chapter 3 offered reflections and exercises to increase awareness and hopefully purge limiting beliefs from your professional lens. Mental health professionals provide a space for individuals to be authentically seen and supported, that allows for vulnerability and reflection. In order to provide this space and this value to clients, we must have language, skills, education, and self-awareness. Our fast-paced world requires constant education. By the time this book is published, terminology may have changed and new skills for supporting clients may have been developed. It is our ethical obligation to remain informed.

Gender Diversity

Gender is diverse and uniquely defined. Gender diversity is an umbrella term representing the diversity of gender expression beyond the binary framework. Terminology discussed within gender diversity includes:

> **Gender**: the attitudes, feelings, and behaviors that are culturally created and associated with a person's biological sex.

DOI: 10.4324/9781003166382-13

Gender-normative means that behaviors are compatible with cultural expectations.

Gender non-conforming is behavior that does not align with the cultural expectations of that gender.

Gender Expression: gender is expressed in physical appearance that communicates gender or gender role. Gender expression may be different from gender identity.

Gender Identity: an internal sense of being as boy, man, girl, woman, genderqueer or nonconforming. It may not correspond with a person's sex assigned at birth. (apa.org)

Gender non-binary describes someone who does not identify exclusively as a man or a woman. Non-binary people may identify as being both a man and a woman, somewhere in between or as falling completely outside these categories.

Transgender describes someone whose gender identity and/or expression is different from cultural expectations based on the sex they were assigned at birth.

Cisgender describes someone whose gender identity aligns with the sex assigned to them at birth (Pleak, 2011).

An awareness of terminology and respect for identity, an individual's pronouns and expressed name are a terrific starting point. The legal name, often associated with insurance or other documents, can feel harmful to the client. Offering space in clinical paperwork as well as initial interaction to correctly name and identify the client is very important.

It is crucial to understand the diversity of treatment interventions for gender non-binary, non-conforming, and transgender individuals. The World Professional Organization of Transgender Health (WPATH) offers a standard of care for transsexual, transgender, and non-conforming people. This standard of care clarifies that not all individuals identifying as transsexual, transgender, and non-conforming experience gender dysphoria, and those that do require individualized therapeutic interventions. It is important for clinicians to remember that identity may not be the presenting problem and although it is important to respect and validate identity, it may not be the primary topic of therapy.

Gender dysphoria is sometimes, certainly not always, a diagnosis or presenting concern for transgender and gender non-binary clients. It is an incorrect assumption that gender dysphoria occurs for every individual in this population. The diagnosis of gender dysphoria to confirm medical necessity for hormone therapy or gender-affirming therapy is often viewed as disempowering for clients. It is often viewed as a form of gatekeeping and decreases access to medical services for clients that may not have resources to access therapy (Florence, 2019). Psychotherapy interventions directly related to gender identity may include exploring identity, role, expression; addressing oppression and discrimination, alleviating internalized transphobia, increasing family, and social support and improving body image (Coleman et al., 2012).

Mental health services for transgender and gender non-binary individuals should address collective trauma. Acknowledgement of discrimination, microaggressions, and threats of or actual violence, as well as trauma-informed modalities to process the experiences, is a necessary element of therapy. The increased symptoms of suicide, suicide ideation, self-harm, substance use disorder, and depression experienced by transgender and gender non-binary population is a result of oppression, discrimination, and minority stress (Brown et al., 2022). The Minority Stress Model is defined by stressors that are unique (not experienced by the non-stigmatized populations), chronic (related to social and cultural structures) and socially based (social processes, institutions, and structures) (Salomaa et al., 2022).

Mental health professionals must also be educated about the diversity of ways individuals live as, or experience transition, as a trans or gender non-conforming individual. It is important to be aware of specific terminology. There are different types of transition or living within your gender identity.

Social transition that includes gender role confirmation, physical expression of gender identity such as clothing, hair, binding (breasts), packing (crotch) and name or pronoun confirmation. For some individuals that are transgender and gender non-confirming, the social transition allows them to live fully in their gender identity (Turban, 2021).

Hormone Therapy

Some individuals may choose hormone therapy in their transition. It is important to note that not all transgender individuals elect hormone therapy. There are biological changes that will occur almost immediately and some changes that will occur over the course of several years. Hormone therapy can result in positive and sometimes negative emotional changes. Support to adjust to changes is an important element of therapy as well as partner, peer or family support during transition. Biological changes include:

MtF (the male to female transition) includes the use of Estrogen and possibly the addition of Progesterone. Changes will include the decrease of facial hair, increase of breast tissue, redistribution of body fat, decreased libido, testicular atrophy, loss of spontaneous erections.

FtM (the female to male transition) includes the use of Testosterone. Changes will include the end of menstruation, facial, and body hair growth, voice deepening, body fat redistribution, clitoral enlargement, vaginal atrophy, possible increase in libido.

(Harris et al., 2022)

Top Surgery

Some transgender and gender non-binary individuals will elect to have top surgery. This includes:

(FtM) Top surgery for transgender men and nonbinary people is a procedure to remove breast or chest tissue (subcutaneous mastectomy). It's also called masculinizing chest surgery.

(MtF) Top surgery for transgender women and nonbinary people is a procedure to increase breast size and change the shape of the chest. It's also called feminizing breast surgery, breast augmentation, chest construction or breast mammoplasty.

These are major surgeries with a month-plus of healing required. Support for the medical and emotional transition is required. Even though this is an "elective" surgery and in most cases offers significant improvement to the reduction of gender dysphoria, if it exists, it is still an adjustment. Any transition, particularly significant changes to the body, requires space to process the change and support.

Bottom Surgery

Some transgender and gender non-binary individuals may elect to have bottom surgery.

(MtF) An individual who decides to have bottom surgery will need to decide between a vaginoplasty or vulvaplasty. The vaginoplasty is more invasive and creates a new opening for the urethra as well as a new opening for the vagina. The creation of a clitoris from the tissue of the penis is also completed during the surgery. The vulvaplasty focuses on the creation of the external vulvar tissue and clitoris, without a vaginal opening. There is less risk with a vulvaplasty but penetrative sex through a vagina is not possible. Both surgeries utilize the tissue of the penis to create the clitoris allowing for orgasmic possibility post-surgery. Recovery requires the on-going use of a dilator to create and maintain depth of the vagina. (Freek et al., 2021)

(FtM) Bottom surgery for individuals having female-to-male gender-affirming surgery includes metoidioplasty and phalloplasty. After the clitoris is enlarged from hormone therapy a metoidioplasty can create a penis from existing tissue. Often referred to as "meta," this penis can obtain an erection. Phalloplasty is more invasive and involves the creation of a penis and urethra from existing skin in other parts of the body. (Freek et al., 2021)

Supporting Adjustment

The changes occurring to the body may be euphoric, overwhelming or there may be feelings of loss. Learning how to interact with one's body as it changes is a process. If someone is partnered or dating, communicating about changes and your body can be an important experience. The therapeutic space can provide room for acknowledging difficulties and celebrating exciting changes. Some of these details may not be topics that are easily covered with friends and family, so the space to acknowledge excitement, difficulty, and possibly feelings of loss, is very useful.

Intersex

Intersex is a socially constructed category used to describe an individual born with reproductive and sexual anatomy that doesn't fit typical definitions of male or female. In medical terminology, Disorders of Sex Development (DSD) is used to describe these differences to internal and/or external anatomy. Some of these differences are apparent at birth such as a scrotum that is very divided and may look more like a labia. Some differences are not identified until puberty or thereafter. DSD can be a harmful term for intersex individuals because it notes something wrong or disordered. Historically, the medical profession often encouraged families to "choose" to identify the child a certain sex based on ways they could make the child "pass." This practice was referred to as the Optum of Gender Rearing and started being practiced in the 1950s. Often this occurred by surgically modifying genitalia of an infant. Families were encouraged to keep this a secret from others, including the child (Bennecke et al., 2021).

The intersex community has worked tirelessly to advocate for an end to surgeries on children's genitals and a discontinuation of the Optum of Gender Rearing medical practice. Male and female is socially constructed and exists on a continuum versus a binary. Intersex individuals do not need to be "fixed" in any way. There is significant psychological harm that has occurred as a result of medical procedures that follow rigid definitions of body standards and sex (Behrens, 2020).

Sexual Orientation

Sexual orientation refers to the pattern of romantic and/or sexual attraction towards others of the same, other or any combination of genders or orientations. Some people might oversimplify sexual orientation as gay or straight. There are actually more than a hundred titles to describe orientations, both romantic and sexual. Sex researcher Alfred Kinsey developed the Kinsey Scale in the late 1940s. The research supports the idea of sexual orientation as a continuum versus a strict binary. Kinsey also suggested sexual orientation was a pattern that was fluid over time. Researcher, author, and psychologist Lisa Diamond also supports this idea of orientation fluidity. Her current research and publications, which primarily focuses on women and sexual orientation, discuss sexual orientation as often fluctuating over the lifespan. In contrast to the notion that bisexuality is "a phase," Diamond's longitudinal research of 79 women points to the existence of orientations beyond simply gay or straight. Terminology may be overwhelming for some but offers important descriptions of romantic and sexual preferences that invites diversity of experience and expression (Diamond, 2008).

Sexual Identity and Expression

"Kink" is an umbrella term that encompasses fetishism, role play, body modification, and BDSM (bondage and discipline, dominance, and submission, sadism and masochism). Broadly, kink represents behaviors that don't align with the social majority. Clients who identify as kinky often face stigma and discrimination. Therapeutic and medical services have historically been viewed as unsafe and pathologizing for kink individuals. Discomfort and lack of information about the kink sexual expression, kink identity, and the kink community has resulted in many mental health professionals expressing discomfort, attempting to analyze or "fix" them (Hansen-Brown & Jefferson, 2022).

There is an important balance of offering a welcoming approach and presenting as educated related to kink identity without placing unwanted attention on kink identity. It is unnecessary and problematic to focus on kink-related topics when the client has not associated it with presenting concerns. Historically, mental health professionals have sought to explore the motivation associated with kink expression, based on their own belief that it must be "caused" by something, rather than simply existing as normal and healthy for their client. The belief that kink is caused by a history of trauma is also incorrect and harmful. It associates kink as something problematic that needs to be healed rather than an individual's unique sexual expression that can be celebrated (New et al., 2021).

BDSM (bondage and discipline, dominance, and submission, sadism, and masochism) includes scenes, roleplays, and props that allow for sexual fantasy that focuses on bondage, restraining or being restrained; dominance, being dominated or submitting control; sadomasochism, inflicting or receiving physical pain or humiliation that is pleasurable. Individuals that participate in BDSM sexual experiences follow the guidelines of safe, sane, and consensual (SSC) or risk aware consensual kink (RACK). Both ideas highlight the importance of individuals having full awareness of the activities and consenting to the activities fully. SSC suggests that there is not risk, thus the safe in the acronym and RACK suggests that risky behavior is permissible of parties are fully aware of the risks (Ling et al., 2022).

Exploration of BDSM should always include an exploration of interests. Discussing interests may include a continuum of "I want to do this, very excited" to "this is interesting, but I'm not sure" to hard limit, "I won't do this." Consent and boundaries should guide each experience. Consent must be very specific to roles, behaviors, and limits. The use of safe words, negotiated before an experience or scene, ensures that individuals can stop even when bondage, domination or pain may be an intentional part of the act. In the last decade, BDSM became a somewhat normalized and exciting term in pop-culture. Movies and books don't necessarily offer details on steps to ensure a consensual experience or represent BDSM accurately. Sexual health advocacy can include information about RACK as well as exploration of interests and practice communicating limits and boundaries (Ling et al., 2022).

Polyamory

Polyamory is a form of consensual non-monogamy that involves multiple adults in relationships with an emphasis on love and emotional intimacy. Sexual intimacy may also be part of polyamorous relationships but is not the emphasis. Polyamorous relationships are configured in many forms. A polycule is a term to describe the network of people in the relationship. Common configurations include but are not limited to:

Vee: one person who is dating two people, those two people are not sexually involved with each other

Triad: three people all involved with each other

Quad: four people that could be two couples or a triad + one person

The management of the polycule can be quite different as well. This includes:

Hierarchical Poly: one relationship is of primary importance over others in the polycule

Non-hierarchical Poly: No relationship is prioritized within the polycule

Solo Poly: an individual in the polycule is not obligated to any partners

Kitchen Table Poly: Focus on family and support not sex or romance although it may exist it is not priority

Parallel Poly: No emotional involvement with others in the polycule beyond primary person

Mono Poly: one person identifies as poly and the other person in the partnership is monogamous

Open Relationships are also consensually non-monogamous; however, the focus is less on emotional intimacy and focused more on sexual intimacy.

Despite terminology becoming more commonly used in our society, individuals in open and polyamorous relationships are often marginalized and misunderstood. Discrimination continues to exist in institutions and in legal protection. Research references mental health practitioners often being uninformed about poly or viewing it as a form of infidelity. Individuals in polyamorous relationships benefit from a mental health professional who demonstrates understanding of consensual non-monogamy and the benefits. The support in exploring the benefits as well as challenges of decision-making, conflict resolution, time management, and communication within a polycule is considered an important part of the therapeutic space (Henrich & Trawinski, 2016).

What Does This Mean About Sex?

There is very little that actually defines what sex is, what it should mean for people, how it should feel, who it should be done with, what makes it successful. This is certainly a message that should sound familiar by this chapter of the book. It is especially important to state this again. The dominant culture sets standards for what is defined as "good," healthy, "normal." This is usually based not on standards of wellness but is rather based on the opinions and power of the dominant culture. This plays out in most things in our culture including, beauty, family practices, language, and of course, sex. Mental health clinicians are often restrained by these limited standards of sex.

The rules and norms that media, parents, religious spaces and health classes handed us must be placed to the side so that we can reimagine the idea of sexuality, sexual expression as unique to each person that enters the therapeutic space. So, here are some new rules:

> Some women have penises.
>
> Some Cis/Het men have sex with men.
>
> Gay men might be a middle and never enjoy penetrating or receiving penetration.
>
> A flaccid penis might be just as fun and sexy as an erect penis.
>
> Successful relationships include people with many partners and isn't infidelity.

We Need to Throw Out Some Ideas

> Sex does not equal penetration.
>
> Erection and lubrication do not equal arousal.
>
> Orgasm does not always involve genitals.

What Is Sex?

Here are some questions we should ask all of our clients, especially transgender and gender non-binary clients:

> What names do you like to use for your "sex parts," or genitals, chest, anus?
>
> Have you ever communicated this with a partner? Do you feel nervous or fearful about that?
>
> What is sex for you?
>
> What warms you up? Or What is foreplay for you?
>
> Do you feel comfortable talking about your body and what it needs before becoming sexually involved with someone?
>
> Do you know how to satisfy yourself and have you ever described that to someone else?

Sex for Transgender Folx

When discussing this topic, it is dangerous to assume that all transgender individuals have sex in monolithic ways. There is a danger in not discussing the topic of transgender sex, that replicates most general sex education and only discusses pronouns and hormones and leaves out sex. Seeking research on the topic of sex for transgender and non-binary folx is a bit complicated. Researchers, educators, allies, doctors, and therapists talk about a lot of other things quite often, but not sex. Publications, documentaries, trainings, and videos focus on topics of pronouns, transition, oppression, and discrimination. There is also the belief that trans bodies are trying to look or behave like cis bodies. It is hard to find the material about trans folx and sex. There is pornography, but there is a standard of fetishizing trans bodies and trans sex in pornography that keeps us from seeing or talking about the real topic. I am approaching this topic with my trans clients in mind, considering what do they need me to know and what issues about sex they want to discuss.

Trans people may have sex with other trans people, or they may have sex with cisgender people. Some trans folx having sex with other trans folx may experience a sense of liberation or celebration of their bodies. There is less often an obligation to "explain" about one's body or sex with one's body when it is "T4T." T4T refers to the dating preference of trans folx exclusively dating other trans folx.

Transgender people dating cisgender people sometimes experience discomfort or frustration due to the explanation that is often required of them to initiate sex. There is also sometimes nervousness about revealing your body to someone who may not know what to expect. Consider a trans woman who has had top surgery, not bottom surgery. She is dating a cisgender woman. There may be anxiety or fear about revealing her body to her new partner. How will her partner react when she sees what is often referred to as a penis? She will have to explain to her cisgender partner what to call her body because she never uses the word "penis." She also will have to explain to her how to touch her body and words to use for specific sex acts. All of this can feel like work. It also comes with apprehension. There may be fear of rejection. For many there is a fear of violence. Violence towards trans bodies, especially related to sex, is horridly very common.

The liberation that some transgender folx discuss about sex is the liberation of being fully seen by another and feeling safe and sexy. It can also be described as the liberation of shedding the limitations and expectations of "cis sex." For most trans children and adolescents there is an "othering," an attempt to fit in or adapt, that is often met with rejection or self-denial. The liberation of not trying, or even wanting to fit inside the limited ideas of gender, also extends to sex. Depending on an individual's transition, they may be fully liberated from the norms and rules of "cis sex," or somewhere in that process. As mental health professionals we can seek to understand that liberation as well as support it.

Transgender sex and cisgender sex both have the potential to be expansive. We can use all the tools we have discussed in this book to support sexual exploration and pleasure. Some specific considerations when working with transgender individuals:

- What you name sexual body parts is largely connected to empowerment.
- What sex acts are called is often different than a cisgender explanation. For example, a transwoman may have what is medically referred to as a penis, but which she calls a "cunt" and refers to oral sex as "eating her out."
- Penetration is not always as valued as in dominant culture.

If you are a cisgender professional reading this book, it might be a good idea to simply remove all the assumptions you hold for sex right now. Place them to the side. Take a breath and feel refreshed. Sex doesn't need to be the way we were told it had to be.

As mental health professionals we must express interest in understanding and exploring the domain of sexuality without pathologizing or fetishizing. If we remove the assumptions, we must be willing to ask open-ended questions about sexual needs, fears, and hopes. Some of the same skills and interventions discussed in Chapter 11 will be useful in this exploration.

Naming, an intervention to empower and encourage communication about the body, is particularly useful for trans clients. We can approach this intervention in a similar manner as described in Chapter 11. Mental health professionals should be particularly thoughtful to listen and ask permission to mirror the language used by the individual for their bodies. Educate yourself and others that are in your network of referrals to avoid gender-laden names for body parts such as breasts or vagina and instead use broad terminology such as chest or genitals. Remember that anatomy and identity are separate. "Pregnant women or prostate exams for men" is incorrect, limiting, and leaves many intersex, transgender, and non-binary people out of the conversation. This can also result in trans, non-binary and intersex individuals not being included in research or being included in necessary information and procedures for their bodies (Green & Maurer, 2015).

The best practices of mental health services allow individuals to speak about symptoms and difficulties without becoming a diagnosis. We help people imagine well-being and healing and then create changes in their resources and support to live into those possibilities. In the same way, sexuality must go beyond the conceptual. When we limit topics to keeping parts healthy, e.g. condoms and STIs, or how to make parts work, we remain outside the actual experience of pleasure, intimacy, and embodiment. Mira Bellwether, author of the zine *Fucking a Trans Woman*, warns of the over-thinking or over-communication about bodies and sex. In an interview with *Autostraddle* she describes, "the more preoccupied or even obsessed you are with the ways in which you are NOT connecting with your body, the less you will be able to enjoy or even experience the ways in which you DO connect with your body." [Trans women sometimes think] about the body in an "instrumental way, like something you are piloting rather than being in, of, a part of" (Kennedy, 2013).

As clinicians discussing well-being, bodies, and intimacy, we need to provide a different type of experience. Visualization activities can give permission to imagine in a safe space and with creative energy. Here is a simple example of beginning the visualization:

- Ask the client to sit comfortably and if they feel safe close their eyes. If that doesn't feel safe, they might find an area of the space to focus their gaze.
- "Become comfortable in your seat and take some slow, deep breaths."

- "Notice your body and focus on an area that feels safe, calm or without discomfort."
- "Allow yourself to visualize a part of you that would like to be touched in a way that brings pleasure. This touch may be yourself or someone else. Picture the rhythm of the touch, the pressure. Can you visualize the response of your body or perhaps a facial expression or sound that expresses your pleasure?"
- "Stay present in this moment."

Certainly, this visualization could be extended to notice feeling in the body, imagine use of words, or extend the vision. I recommend beginning simply followed by processing the experience. The focus is to help the individual become present to themselves and the idea of sexual pleasure without the responsibility of communicating. Note the element of visualizing themselves as feeling pleasure whether in a facial expression or maybe a sound. Viewing one's self as sexy, erotic, is an important element of pleasure. This is important for all people. It is especially important for trans and non-binary individuals because they have less representations of their bodies as sexy and beautiful without being fetishized. This part of the visualization also embraces the fluidity of erotic expression in constant state of change and development.

Communication

The use of Body Maps and Mindful Touch interventions may aid in individual or couples' communication of sexual needs, boundaries, limits, pleasure, and safety. Special attention should be placed on types of touch and words to use to describe this with partners. Depending on the needs of the client, these interventions may focus more on sexual health and communication or more on pleasure and sexual embodiment. A lot of pressure is placed on transgender and gender non-binary individuals to name and describe their bodies in medical settings and with partners. This is an important element of safety and empowerment. Body Maps and Mindful Touch also allow clients to feel about their bodies in a new way that is curious and sexy. Be thoughtful in guiding the exercises based on the needs of your client.

Here is a case example that illustrates some of the concepts discussed in this chapter.

Case Example – Nova

Nova is a transgender man who began social transition at age 25. He started seeing his social worker at age 20 years old. He had socially transitioned in employment and with family and friends. He had survived some losses due to coming out, including his best friend, an uncle and grandfather that no longer spoke to him. The majority of friends and family were informed and supportive.

He had recently started dating. He felt excited about her. She identified as cisgender and was aware of his identity as a transgender man. Nova wanted to be in a sexual relationship with his new girlfriend but struggled to communicate about how he wanted to be sexual and worried that the sex might not be fulfilling to his new partner.

Nova had two goals to work on in therapy. The first goal was to feel comfortable with his body. The second goal was communicating about sexuality with his new partner. Nova was invited to complete the Naming intervention and very quickly noticed a disconnect or feeling "sterile" as he discussed parts of his body. I challenged him to change his tone and inflection to represent the feeling associated with different parts. I also challenged him to imagine introducing these parts to someone new in a way that described the feeling about the parts. Nova noticed a lot of emotions surfacing with these challenges. He noticed that some words he had adopted because he had heard others use the terms and he decided during the exercise, these terms didn't fit. For instance, he used the word "dick" but felt that the way he wanted to be touched on this part of him didn't resonate with the word "dick." He tried on different terms and allowed himself to be playful with the process.

Nova had top surgery during the time he was in therapy. He felt excited to sit in his bed or watch television with his shirt off but was also a bit anxious. When he brought this up in therapy, I offered the visualization as a way to explore. He noted that during the visualization the feeling of anxiety was very present initially and then was replaced by a feeling of sexiness and excitement. During the following week he tried out being in his home alone with his top off and reported feeling "pure joy" in these moments. He expressed that he wanted to take his shirt off in front of his partner but worried that she might be distracted by his scars from top surgery. I reframed this, "I wonder if you might feel fixated on the scars and are projecting this on to her?" He took a photo of his chest and placed it in a journal. I encouraged him to take a look at the photo a few times a day and write words in the journal that came to mind. Nova returned the next week and shared the journal. Listening to him read the words, a wave of change occurred from beginning to end. "Pain, raw, scared" were words at the beginning and towards the end, "lifeline, new, tough." He expressed feeling more ready to be seen by his partner.

Nova spent a month in therapy expressing excitement over his relationship with his partner. They were spending a lot of time together. Anxiety and uncertainty surrounding their sexual relationship surfaced as the relationship progressed.

Nova wanted to progress to receiving oral sex, perhaps have penetrative anal sex and maybe a "hand job." He felt overwhelmed by the fear of rejection from his partner even though he couldn't identify anything she had expressed that made him feel this would occur. During sessions we modified the visualization exercise to help him picture them lying beside each other naked. We repeated the visualization several times within sessions and this allowed Nova to progress through emotions of fear and some shame that he held. Eventually, we completed the visualization which was always very similar,

- Ask the client to sit comfortably and if they feel safe close their eyes. If that doesn't feel safe, they might find an area of the space to focus their gaze.
- "Become comfortable in your seat and take some slow, deep breaths."
- "Notice your body and focus on an area that feels safe, calm or without discomfort."
- "(1) Allow yourself to visualize your partner enjoying being beside you naked. (2) Allow yourself to visualize your partner smiling as she looks at you in front of her (3) Allow yourself to visualize a part of you that would like to be touched in a way that brings pleasure. This touch may be yourself or someone else. Picture the rhythm of the touch, the pressure. Can you visualize the response of your body or perhaps a facial expression or sound that expresses your pleasure?"
- "Stay present in this moment."

Nova opened his eyes and smiled. After several weeks of practicing the visualization the feelings of shame and fear resolved and "sexy" was the word that came to mind as he opened his eyes. Nova and his partner began to explore more sexual intimacy together. In session, we discussed language a lot and practicing ways to communicate touch and movement that didn't "ruin the mood" but still felt consensual and safe. Nova and his partner were sexually informed about one another's bodies and sexually creative because they allowed themselves to be centered in their own experiences. Nova moved from thinking about his body to imagining, visualizing, knowing it, feeling it.

As you conclude reading this chapter, I hope you have been able to give yourself permission to be curious, adaptive, and creative about sex. This work is not about trying to get it right but making space for "right" to be unique and expansive.

Questions for Reflection and Discussion

When you consider challenging perspectives of family members or partners about what sex should be or can be, what do you imagine you will encounter? How will you respond? What is the balance of challenge and compassion?

Aging and Sexual Expression

13

The aging population, or retirement population, is the fastest growing sector in the United States. A gradual reduction in the stigma of mental health services is resulting in more older adults accessing a mental health professional, more now than any time in history. Awareness of common presenting concerns is useful for therapists.

Aging presents gradual stages of transition in multiple domains of individuals' lives. Family structures change including relatives aging and perhaps requiring more care, while children are often producing their own children and moving out of the home. Employment may change based on the type of work an individual can maintain. Individuals that have used their body for employment may need to transition to a different type of work. Some individuals may choose to retire, resulting in excess time in their personal life. This is lonely and overwhelming for many individuals. Aging individuals in long-term relationships may have grown away from one another over many years in a relationship. Often resentments in relationships have gone unaddressed due to lack of knowledge or time to resolve problems. Past losses and traumas often resurface in older age. Bodies change in ability and appearance. Many experience increased medical issues, a need for more medication or more medical care.

Sexual expression and relationships are influenced by all of these changes. With support, resources, and psychoeducation, individuals may have more time and energy to focus on their sexual selves and experience. There is the potential for more pleasure in this era of their lives than ever before. Without the support, resources, and psychoeducation, increased sexual problems of

DOI: 10.4324/9781003166382-14

pain, avoidance, and frustration will often overtake the possibility of pleasure and sexual transition (Taylor & Gosney, 2011).

Biological Transition

The biological female body is affected by the decline in estrogen and progesterone over the course of perimenopause and menopause. This results in changes to menstruation and eventual end to the menstrual cycle. Changes in sleep, hot flashes, fatigue, irritability, and vaginal dryness are directly related to the reduction of estrogen and progesterone.

The biological male body experiences a slower decline of testosterone over time. Beginning around age 30, testosterone levels decrease at approximately 1% each year. This build-up of consistent loss may affect penis erections, both in obtaining and maintaining, and degree of rigidity of erection.

Psychological Transition

The hormonal changes that occur rather dramatically for biological females, due to the decrease in estrogen and progesterone, can cause irritability, decreased energy, low mood or sadness. Similar to puberty, perimenopause, and menopause are times of transition in an individual's life. Not only does the person need to adjust to changes in how their body looks and feels, they often experiences changes in social and relational experiences and expectations. As mental health professionals we can normalize the significance of aspects of aging on the body and also help clients be thoughtful about this phase of their life. Increasing resources and support in their environment and for their body is useful. Helping clients lean into the possibility that exists in change and listening more intently to how they feel can help clients to embrace this phase rather than regret or deny changes. Sometimes changes are experienced as loss. There may be increased symptoms of depression, as well as experiences of grief.

The adjustment to how the body performs and feels also may cause feelings of loss. Being able to help individuals interpret the messages of their body and energy and set new expectations in their lifestyle that align with these changes is important. Aging in mid-life, as well as senior years, can offer an opportunity for reflection. It Is common for a resurfacing of challenging times. This can be confusing to individuals because they may feel they have already "dealt with these things." Meaning-making occurs across the lifespan.

As we develop and gain wisdom, we have new tools to make sense of earlier experiences. Helping clients embrace this opportunity for meaning-making, and possibly changing their narrative about an experience, can be very beneficial.

Many individuals will face health concerns in their older years. Increased anxiety related to health problems often surface and require therapeutic attention. Depression related to medical concerns is also common. When medical problems become the central focus, considering diseases like cancer, the individual may feel that they have lost control over autonomy. Another common feeling is that they have lost the ability to be seen as a whole person and are only perceived related to their diagnosis. The decreased functioning of their bodies when severe medical diagnoses exist can also intrude in the possibility of engaging in social and personal domains that brought meaning to the client's life.

Changes in identity can also be overwhelming. Mid-life and senior years are filled with transitions of employment, children moving into adulthood, changing home environments, and these are just a few considerations. Moving through these transitions requires reflecting on the meaning, grieving the losses, in order to open to change. Sometimes when individuals do not have support, the reflection and grieving do not occur and they are paused in a space in time. It is common that adjustment disorders and depression diagnoses may be common.

Depression may be associated with any and all of these issues. Major Depressive Disorder or Persistent Mood Disorder have symptoms of decreased pleasure, sad mood, lowered energy, all of which impact relationships and sexual functioning.

Relational Transition

The idea of long-term mates that are attachment as well as romantic and sexual partners is a fairly new phenomenon in the course of history. Psychotherapist and author Ester Perel states, "today, we turn to one person to provide what an entire village once did: a sense of grounding, meaning, and continuity. At the same time, we expect our committed relationships to be romantic as well as emotionally and sexually fulfilling. Is it any wonder that so many relationships crumble under the weight of it all?" (Perel, Mating in Captivity). Individuals in long-term relationships will not only need to weather all these transitions together, they will likely also have to consider if the person they are becoming is suited for the person their partner is becoming. It is expected, necessary, and unavoidable that we change intellectually, emotionally, physically, and relationally as we grow and age. It is possibly a slight miracle we can align these changes with the partner we may have started with 25–50 years previously. Therapy can be a space to contemplate this alignment or possibly apply strategies to heal or challenge relational dynamics.

For individuals who are not in long-term relationships, they face new challenges related to the transition of aging. Navigating changes to the body, changes to how we want to be sexual, while dating, can be intimidating. Commonly, individuals avoid dating due to feeling intimidated or uncertain how to communicate about changes. Decreased confidence and uncertainty may result in individuals fixating on certain aspects of themselves. Modifications that change the appearance of the body, or adaptations to the body, that aid sexual performance are often associated with adapting to dating while aging. Helping clients think about long-term goals for pleasure and relationships is important.

Loss of a partner is an unfortunate and common reality of aging. Grief and loss are important elements of therapy. They may lead to guilt or fear of beginning a new relationship. Contemplating a new relationship after a long-term relationship has ended can be very scary. Considerations of pacing the relationship as well as emotional, sexual, and physical safety are helpful to explore in therapy. Helping the client by practicing communicating through psychoeducation or roleplay is very useful.

Divorce during mid-life may be a time that individuals enter therapy. In some way they may be experiencing a death of their relationship and way of life. Individuals who may have prompted the divorce may feel blamed or guilty. Sometimes, individuals felt that they had no choice and were dumped or left behind. This can be especially complicated if there is a known affair. There is the loss of a family for this couple as well. This is made even more difficult if they are trying to learn to co-parent children or care for pets and extended family through this process. There is often a feeling of responsibility to other family members. It is important to validate their sense of concern or guilt, make space for the grief and loss and help establish responsibility for the things within their control and give back other responsibilities to those in their lives that may be surprised or hurt from the separation or divorce.

Sexual Transition

Changes to a person's sexual expression and experience is a culmination of all the factors we have thus far discussed in this chapter. When individuals experience many changes in their lives they may want to hold on to consistency in areas of life that they are able to do so. Finding spaces that pleasure feels predictable can be comforting and reassuring. This might be in ways that they express themselves as sexy and feel positive or maybe it is how they masturbate. It is also important to name this time as a space of change, transition, and work to frame it with the client as an opportunity. In earlier stages of life, individuals did not have the same amount of knowledge about their bodies or sexual interests as they do in mid-life or senior years. This knowledge is wisdom and in the space of mental health services we can help them identify new needs and wants. Exploring what could be possible and how to look for that and ask for that, is clarifying and empowering (Ratner et al., 2011).

In order to recognize difficulties experienced in sexual transition or sexual developmental change, professionals need to be familiar with common presenting problems.

Common Problems in Mid-Life (45–65 Years of Age)

Pain and Sex

The decrease of estrogen and progesterone results in a decrease in vaginal lubrication as well as vaginal atrophy, a thinning, drying, and inflammation of the vaginal walls. Untreated, this can cause pain with any form of penetration. It may also cause discomfort due to itching and tightness even without penetration. Pain during penetrative sex is described as dyspareunia. It refers to painful vaginal sex either at the introitus, or opening of the vagina, or deep in during penetration and thrusting during sex. The decrease in estrogen during menopause can sometimes lead to urinary problems. Pain may also be caused by pelvic injury from childbirth or from scarring associated with surgery or radiation treatment.

Addressing vaginal atrophy, thinning, and drying of vaginal walls is a very important part of treatment. Even in cases when a person with a vagina does not choose to have penetrative sex, wellness for the vagina requires care for this part of the body. Lubrication that can be used daily can aid in sexual activities as well as a daily lubricant. There are many different types of lubricants, like water-based, silicone-based and oil-based lubricants. Water-based can be used with all condoms and all sex toys. It does not last quite as long as other types of lubricants. Silicone-based lubricants are more slippery and last longer. They can be more difficult to clean from material such as bed sheets or clothing. They can be used with condoms but may degrade sex toys. Oil-based lubricants such as Vaseline, olive oil or vitamin E will degrade condoms or toys. There is also the risk of increasing infection because they leave a coating that traps bacteria.

In addition to the use of lubrication, moisture for the vagina is also very important. A low-dose estrogen therapy that is vaginally inserted in the form of a cream, vaginal tablet or flexible vaginal ring provides a reversal of changes to vaginal tissue caused by menopause. The risk associated with estrogen exposure is very low and considered safe by most doctors who will prescribe these forms of vaginal moisturizers. There are also non-estrogen vaginal moisturizers that are applied internally and can provide similar benefits.

Vaginal atrophy should also be addressed with vaginal stretching. With the use of a vaginal moisturizer to repair the lining of the vaginal walls, penetration works to reduce atrophy. If an individual is having penetrative sex with a partner once a week, this can be considered a beneficial therapy to vaginal atrophy. Vaginal dilators, or a sex toy used weekly, can also provide this benefit. This does not have to be considered sexually pleasurable, though it certainly can be. It is truly necessary for the health of the body as it ages (Foley, Kope, Sugrue, 2012).

In a relationship where vaginal and penile penetration is a goal, the use of medication to obtain erection, such as Viagra, Cialis, may be problematic without proper attention to a partner's biological experience. Medications to treat erectile dysfunction are often prescribed with little explanation and little assessment regarding the relational, sexual dynamic. Erections may be more rigid and last longer when assisted by a medication. Penetration can be difficult or painful when hormone levels change. Tearing and fissures can occur in the vagina as a result. The anxiety of pain develops easily and can become a difficult and separate issue.

Erectile Difficulty (ED)

The rigidness and duration of an erection changes over the life course with the natural decrease in testosterone. This certainly does not mean that intimacy needs to end as people age. It does mean that finding new ways to experience intimacy is important as well as understanding the resources for improving the quality or duration of your erection. Adapting sexual behaviors in addition to medical or biological responses allows for continued pleasure and sexual confidence. It is important to discuss sexual pleasure and change directly with clients. Some individuals may feel that they must simply accept that there is less intimacy due to changes in their body. This often results in, distance in relationships and feelings of loss. It is often a contributing factor in depression.

Prostate cancer and its treatment is also associated with erectile difficulty. Most individuals are able to regain erections post treatment, especially with the proper care and treatment advice post-surgery. Nerve-sparing surgery yields positive results for regaining erections within approximately two years of treatment. Hormone therapy for prostate cancer androgen deprivation therapy is used in cases of advanced prostate cancer or when PSA (prostate specific antigen) remains high after initial treatment. There is a correlation with erectile dysfunction and increased suicidal ideation particularly among older adults. For many individuals with a penis, fear about the loss of sexual pleasure and the changes to sexual expression are quite overwhelming. Discussing this issue and how it is being addressed is directly related to mental health.

Treatment Options for Erectile Dysfunction

Oral medications (Viagra, Levitra, Cialis) are often prescribed to address erectile dysfunction. They are most often prescribed by a primary care doctor and often detailed assessment about sexual functioning and intimacy is not addressed. The medications work by increasing the ability to get an erection when sexually stimulated. The increase in nitric oxide relaxes the muscles in the penis allowing blood to flow more freely. Sexual stimulation is still required to allow the medication to work. When factors include psychological or relational difficulties and they go untreated, the medication will have limited effectiveness over the course of several months. Often the initial experiences of erectile difficulty can increase performance anxiety which can create a difficult cycle of: intimacy – performance anxiety – decreased erotic focus – ED. While the medication can treat the biological factors of ED, performance anxiety and lack of focus are psycho-relational issues that are addressed in other ways.

Using some of the treatment techniques in Chapter 11 can help individuals with ED and their partners think about what allows for sexual desire. Being willing to consider new ways to explore intimacy may increase arousal as well as offer a distraction from the ED. Many individuals interpret the loss of an erection as an end to the experience. Help them view this as a pause versus an end and redirect to something else arousing. In a solo sexual experience the individual might stop to fantasize for a few minutes and then return to masturbation. In a partnered experience the individual could focus on touching their partner in a different way or directing touch to a different part of themselves. Often, moving the focus to something else arousing and then returning to a penetrative experience can successfully address performance anxiety. For couples that have been in long-term relationships they may have become very routine in their sexual expression. The introduction of romance in the relationship, toys, erotica or pornography can offer something different and increased desire and focus.

Some individuals may not be able to take oral medication for erectile dysfunction. This includes individuals with hypotension, untreated hypertension, liver or kidney damage, heart disease, sickle-cell anemia, multiple myeloma, and leukemia. A vacuum pump can also aid in having an erection. The vacuum pump, or vacuum constriction device is placed over the penis and the constriction of air pulls blood flow to the penis. This can be done prior to having penetrative sex. It is also used for the health of the penis. If blood flow is restricted, penis pumps or vacuum pumps are recommended to bring increased blood flow to the penis, necessary for the health of tissues in the penis.

Other considerations to address ED include penile injections and penile implants. Penile injections are usually self-administered after first learning in the doctor's office. They are more invasive and for that reason generally not the first consideration. For individuals that cannot be helped by or easily use other methods, penile implants are an option. An erection can be induced by pressing a button installed under the scrotum. This may be a solution for individuals who could not use or were not aided by other medical interventions. This may commonly be the case for individuals with Peyroine's Disease, a painful curvature of the penis.

Many medications prescribed during older years can interfere in sexual functioning and desire.

> **Antidepressants** – used to treat anxiety and depression symptoms and can cause loss or decrease in libido, decreased, or difficulty maintaining arousal, anorgasmia, or reduced quality of orgasm
>
> **Antipsychotics** – used to treat severe mental illness these medications can cause, ED, decreased desire, anorgasmia, or reduced quality of orgasm, retrograde ejaculation, and delayed ejaculation
>
> **Antiandrogens** – used to treat androgen-dependent diseases and causes suppression of desire, arousal, and orgasm.
>
> **Immunosuppressants** – steroids used to treat chronic inflammatory diseases decrease testosterone and lead to ED

Diuretics – used to treat heart failure, liver failure, and certain kidney disorders may cause which may cause changes to sex hormones as well as ED

HIV Meds – increase in ED over the course of treatment

Antiepileptic Drugs – disruption in sex hormone levels and decreased libido

Dopamine Agonist – used in the treatment of Parkinson's Disease can cause heightened libido and hypersexual behavior

Common Problems in Aging or Senior Years (66+)

As people age, they may seek to change their living situation. This decision is often based on the need for additional care and results in an assisted living or nursing facility. Residing in these spaces can result in obstacles to privacy and decision-making regarding sexual expression. Social workers, administrators, and care staff often feel uncomfortable acknowledging sexual health and intimacy with aging clients. They are often pressured by family members that feel sexual behavior of their relative is inappropriate or harmful. This can result in numerous risks for aging clients living in facilities. Lack of information about caring for and protecting their bodies has resulted in increased STIs among aging clients. Lack of education or communication related to consent and decision-making also increases the risk of physical and emotional harm for residents. Privacy that would allow clients to engage safely in sexual experiences with one another or even solo is often restricted.

There are specific concerns and beliefs surrounding the sexuality and intimacy in facilities for aging populations. The belief held by some, that older people are not, or should not be sexual, is often referenced. Although incorrect, it remains an influential belief due to stigma of aging and discomfort with sexuality in general. Concerns related to memory are also referenced as reasons clients should not be sexually active. When autonomy is viewed as a dichotomy versus values, beliefs, and capacity that fluctuates, then rigid rules are upheld for individuals.

An alternative is the idea of "now" person. A "now" person is not a fixed but ever-changing sense of personhood and sexual self that is influenced by environment, relationships, growth, health, and transition. A "then" person is a fixed sense of moral agency of the individual that is set and unchanging in personhood and sexual self. Through direct and on-going conversations with aging clients we can help them assess emotional and physical safety for sexual behavior as well as select some type of intimacy versus entirely restricting it. When sexual expression is completely restricted it limits touch and expression and is harmful emotionally. These forms of connection to one's self and others are especially important and comforting when individuals may be isolated from many comforts they once enjoyed (Sokolowski, 2012).

Direct and on-going conversations help the individual to assess:

- What is the meaning or the relationship or behavior for the client?
- Is there capacity to acknowledge the freedom to decline aspects of the relationship/behavior?
- Is there capacity to contemplate risks/benefits?
- What values are held by the client in making decisions to engage/not engage?

When sexual rights to autonomy and privacy are discussed as part of the mission of the residential facility it provides clarity to staff, residents, and family members. Family members can be encouraged to be part of the conversations with their loved ones, but staff should uphold confidentiality of the residents rather than talk about them with their family. Information about sexual health and care for the residents' health and body can also be openly addressed when the mission of sexual rights and health is made clear in the agency mission.

Case Study: Mitch and Ellie

Mitch is a 75-year-old man who was married for 42 years to the mother of his four children. Shortly after his wife died of ovarian cancer, he broke his hip. After he completed rehab, he exhibited symptoms of depression and often expressed hopelessness when he spoke with his adult children. The home he lived in was too much to care for and he agreed to move into an assisted-care facility.

Ellie is a 74-year-old woman who was married for 40 years. She has one adult daughter. She is a widow. Ellie felt scared to stay alone after her husband died. She wanted more support and protection around her and opted for an assisted living facility.

Mitch and Ellie met in the assisted care facility. Mitch had been there about six months when Ellie moved in. He offered to help show her around and they became fast friends. When Ellie's daughter visited from out of state about three months after she moved into the facility, Elle shared with her that it was exciting to feel "alive again." Ellie referenced her new relationship with Mitch and shared that they sometimes spent the night with one another. Ellie's daughter reacted with anger and concern and told her mother that wasn't "safe or appropriate." Before leaving town, the daughter filed a formal complaint with the social worker, stating that the facility was failing to keep her mother safe.

When Mitch's oldest son visited weekly, he noted how happy his dad had become. They often shared lunch or dinner with Ellie at their table. Mitch noted that sometimes Ellie and his father were forgetful. He felt grateful they were in this safe facility and had each other for companionship. His father noted that it felt so comforting to stay the night beside Ellie. His son understood and was grateful that he had found someone else to share important moments with after the loss of his wife.

The social worker at the facility was contacted by administration and asked to address the "unsafe situation" of Ellie. When she spoke with Ellie, she asked about her relationship with Mitch. Ellie shared that Mitch was the reason she finally felt grateful and happy again. She acknowledged that they did spend the night in each other's rooms. She said that they hadn't had penetrative sex but they did do "lots of other things." The social worker asked Ellie if she had any questions or needed any resources to feel safer and healthier in her relationship. Ellie asked the social worker about precautions against yeast infections or urinary tract infections if they had any type of digital (finger) penetration or oral sex. The social worker provided information about urinating after any type of sexual activity as a natural cleansing practice. Cranberry supplements to aid urinary health was advised. The social worker also explained symptoms of yeast and urinary tract infections and provided individual testing strips that Ellie could use. She explained the use of condoms or dental dams during oral sex and offered to provide them in case they were needed. The social worker reported back to the administration that based on the questions she used to discuss safety and awareness of sexual feelings and behaviors, Ellie was emotionally and physically safe. Although Ellie's daughter was unhappy with this report, she was glad that they had talked to her mother about the relationship. The facility's mission and policies allowed them to prioritize autonomy of the person at the time and acknowledge sexual rights as important to care.

Assisting Clients in Navigating Sexual Transition

The acknowledgement that sexuality traverses the lifespan is an important starting point for individuals seeking mental health services. We acknowledge this in asking direct questions in assessment material. As a clinician, you may feel fearful of offending someone that is older than you by asking questions about their sexuality and sexual experiences. Remember the assessment tools referenced in earlier chapters. Name sexual health and intimacy as an important domain of functioning and move into specific questions and topics.

Focusing on transition for mid-life and aging clients is most important. Transitions in family dynamics, intimate relationships, body image and health changes. All of these influence mental health as well as sexual health and intimacy. Reflection on what was is different from trying to return to something earlier in our experience. These core components may guide us through treatment:

> *Reflection:* Life transitions offer the opportunity to evaluate what has been. This may include celebrations of accomplishments. This may include regrets for things we wish we had done differently. We can prompt this by asking about the "best times" and the "difficult times." More broadly we can ask about the photographs that are most clear in their memory.
>
> *Evaluation of needs*: Recognition of developmental change allows us to reflect on new and different needs and wants. We can help clients by acknowledging needs/wants that were met previously and differentiating from current needs/wants. This helps us to understand that relationships that once met needs may no longer because needs change even when people still care for one another.
>
> *Communication:* Acknowledgement of change requires intrapersonal communication. Helping individuals be honest about what they need and want is a first step. This can be scary for clients to acknowledge because once it is acknowledged it is impossible to unsee it. This prompts change that is often scary. Finding ways to communicate with partners about what they need/want is a second step. Recognizing and preparing for ways that these needs/wants may create conflict, confusion, excitement, change, etc. is also important therapeutic work.

Often what is identified as a 'mid-life crisis,' is a developmental task. It is influenced by hormonal changes discussed earlier in this chapter, as well as psychological and relational changes. As mental health professionals we can help individuals establish routine, balance, and self-care to help them through this developmental stage. We can also help them contemplate the experience they are seeking and meaning associated with this experience. Sometimes clients focus on what they are trying to go away from and benefit from contemplating what they are going toward. When I client focuses a great deal on a job they hate and want to leave or a relationship that is terrible and they want to end, we can challenge them to focus on what they are moving toward. Development stages throughout the life course are often interpreted or understood as a rejection. They can be better understood as a development need of discovery or becoming. If we help clients lean into the meaning of their emotions and behaviors, we can help them make responsible decisions that will best align with their sexual values.

Case Study: Steven

Steven is a 50-year-old cisgender, gay man in a partnered relationship. He and his partner of 20 years have established a sexual relationship that is mostly monogamous and sometimes sexually open. When they open up the relationship it is agreed they will invite the individual into a sexual experience that both know about or both are involved in.

When Steven begins therapy, he describes feeling guilty and uncertain. He is attracted to someone he met at the bar recently. He has been communicating with him quite a bit, with naked pictures and sexting. He hasn't told his partner and he isn't sure that he wants to tell him. I ask him to share a bit about their relationship. He discusses a close emotional relationship with his partner. His partner experienced physical and emotional abuse as a child and came into the relationship with a lot of attachment wounds. Steven has acted as a source of love and support. He expresses that he is grateful for their relationship and everything that they have given to each other but, he also wonders what he would have experienced if the support would have focused on him. (Reflection)

In the last year he has been a source of support for his brother in substance use recovery program. He has reflected a great deal on the relationship with this mother and his role in the family of origin. He shares with me that he is always the person in control, the caretaker and wishes he could finally let go. He became aware of this deep desire when he was dancing with this new person at the bar and wanted just "be free." He states, "this is sexual for sure, but also about my role in all my relationships. I want to feel free and I don't think I can do that with Dan" [is partner]. (Evaluation of needs)

I ask Steven to simply listen to what he is saying. I repeat back to him his phrase, "I want to be free." I ask him to describe what that feels like. He begins to tell me, and I ask him to simply tell himself. He sits upright and with a firmer voice says, "I need to be able to be weak and be loved. I want to feel sexy when I am weak and vulnerable. I am so tired of always being the strong one." He begins to cry and then finally smiles. I nod and acknowledge, "I think you know what you need." (Communication)

In our next session, I challenge Steven to consider communicating as openly with Dan as he has with himself. At first, he considers ignoring his needs and wants. Then he switches to his concerns that Dan would be "destroyed" if he shared these feelings. I challenged him to consider the most harmful thing would be putting Dan at emotional or physical risk or breaking trust. Steve cried and acknowledged that he needed to be honest with Dan and he was scared. We began practicing the conversations.

Following the phases of reflection, evaluation, and communication can move individuals from guilt and self-blame to increased insight. It can also help to encourage responsibility to sexual values and away from secrecy and uncertainty.

Conclusion

Sex of all forms has enormous benefits for emotional, relational, and physical health. The experience of desire and arousal associated with sexual experiences generally reduces short-term pain, reduces blood pressure, improves sleep, improves immune system, and helps manage stress. Helping adults find successful and pleasurable ways to be sexual is important to mental and physical well-being. Validating the importance of sexual relationships and offering resources and information to keep bodies safe is core to well-being services. Sexuality and intimacy are core to our sense of humanity throughout the lifespan. Validating the sexual needs and rights of aging adults is core to mental health. Providing education and resources allows them to be sexual in ways that are emotionally and physically safe and pleasurable.

Questions for Reflection and Discussion

What are potential risks for individuals in assisted care or nursing facilities surrounding sexual expression? How do best practices for sexual rights run up against issues of professional liability? How can risks be managed?

Networking, Resources, Referrals, and Coordination of Care

14

Introduction

This chapter will explore the network that every mental health provider should identify and have access to in their community to be responsive to the variety of needs presented by clients. Approaches to find and connect with other helping professionals will be provided. The process of coordinating care for sexual health issues including introducing the process to the client and written documentation with medical, psychiatric, and integrative care specialists.

As mental health professionals we often fill multiple roles in the lives of our clients. Our work includes assessment and diagnosis, creation of treatment plans, support in decision-making, challenging patterns, exploring motivation, psychoeducation, teaching, and providing grounding and mindfulness. In addition, we act as advocates and providers of resources. Resource provision requires, (1) knowing what is needed (2) the development of a network of providers, (3) coordination of care with providers, and (4) introducing the process to the client. This chapter will address all four elements.

Knowing What Is Needed

Being prepared with a referral network ensures that we are able to "stay in our lane" as mental health providers and also be able to help clients address other needs that are outside of our work or expertise. We can use the domains

DOI: 10.4324/9781003166382-15

Family
- **Mental Health**
- **Substance Abuse** ⟶
- **Abuse/Neglect**
- Inter-generational Responsibilities

Health
- **Medication**
- Medical Problem
- **Sexual Pain** ⟶
- Fertility
- **Sexual Difficulty**
- Nutrition
- **Substance Abuse**
- **Chronic Pain**

Financial / Legal
- Divorce/Custody
- Probation/Parole ⟶
- Bankruptcy
- **Food Stamps – Cash Assistance**
- **Insurance**

AA/NA Groups In-patient Partial Hospitalization Intensive Out-patient Adult/Child Protective Services

Primary Care Psychiatry Gynecology Urology Pelvic Floor Physical Therapy

Department of Health & Human Services Medicare, Medicaid, Commercial Insurances

Education/Employment
- Unemployment
- Job Search ⟶
- Student Loans
- **Educational Accommodations**
- **Short-term/Long-term disability**
- **Family Leave**

Spiritual
- Religious Support ⟶
- Spiritual Exploration
- Healing
- Grieving

Student Services (College/University) Counseling/Social Work (k-12 Schooling) Disability Attorney FMLA Human Resource Departments

Local Religious Institutions Hospice Pastoral Care Programs

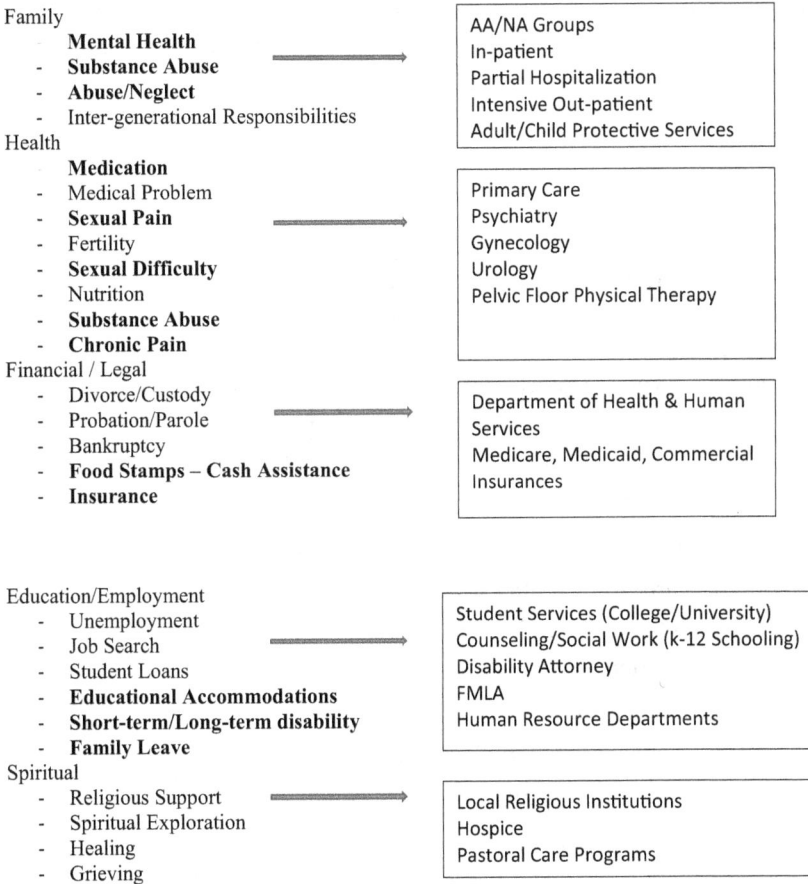

Figure 14.1 Knowing What is Needed: Client Needs and Sources of Referral

of the biopsychosocial to identify what may be needed. On the left are the areas that directly relate to social work. Text in bold identifies areas that often require additional networking or coordination of care. Services/providers on the right we may often network with to address the full range of client issues.

Developing a Network of Providers

When we provide a referral to a service, we should have a clear idea of the process of beginning and receiving services so that we are able to prepare our clients. We can also establish a relationship with the providers to ease the referral process and coordination of care. We should always be clear with clients that they are not required to use the referrals we are providing, rather they are a suggestion.

Beginning the Process

When you are new to the community you will be practicing in, you can ask other trusted mental health workers for suggestions about their referral sources. You might also do an Internet search, speak with community organizations, doctors or speak with the Better Business Bureau. A list of questions to services providers that you are interviewing for your network of referrals:

What is the best way for a new client to access care?

Is there a waitlist for services?

What information or paperwork will a new client need to begin services?

What are the identities held by providers (do they reflect the demographics of the community or your client base)?

Is the location/services ADA compliant/accessible?

What insurances are accepted?

What languages are servcies provided?

Is there a commitment for undocumented/refugee clients?

Do providers share LGBTQIA+ identities and have they received training in LGBTQIA+ informed service provision?

What is the cost for services?

Is there a sliding-scale?

If I am providing a referral what would be helpful information to provide on behalf of my client?

What ages do you provide services for?

If a service provider feels like a good fit for your network it is best practice to introduce yourself, if at all possible, in person. Dropping off your business card or sharing an email introduction with your website link is also useful. Once you have established a network of specialists through which to refer, you can begin coordinating care on behalf of clients.

Coordination of Care

Before you can coordinate care on behalf of your client you will need their permission to share information. You need to document this permission in writing through a Release of Information. The Release of Information should identify:

Client Name

Date of Birth

Information they are agreeing to release

Dates beginning/ending that they are releasing information or expiration of release of information

The place/provider they are releasing information

Client name printed beside the signature

Date of signature

It is important to educate clients on the importance of being very specific about what they agree to release and for a limited amount of time. It is important to protect personal information and not sign-off on more than necessary.

Depending on the need/topic you are seeking to coordinate care for, the information provided will change. As a general rule you should offer limited information and provide your contact information in case they would like to request more information. Here are some suggestions:

With some referral sources your purpose is to introduce the client by name and what is being sought by the referral to their services. This is the case for:

Department of Health and Human Services

AA/NA Groups

With some referral sources you are introducing the client as proof of their participation in services. You should share your client's name, date of birth, how often they participate in therapy and the duration of their time in therapy. This is the case for:

Court

Probation/Parole

Employer

Department of Health and Human Services

With some referral sources you should include the client's name, date of birth, their diagnosis and length of time in treatment services:

Disability attorney

School Social Work or Counselor

Student Accommodations

The most information should be shared when coordinating care for mental health treatment or services related to sexual dysfunction or sexual pain. Provide the client's name, date of birth, reason for referral, current diagnosis, current treatment interventions, symptoms associated with most difficulties and how long symptoms have existed. This includes:

Primary Care Physician

Psychiatry

Gynecology

Urology

Pelvic Floor Physical Therapy

Chapter 11 provided information about how specific health concerns are treated by specific specialists.

Connecting With Community Support

When you have trusted sources of support in the community that can be useful to clients but may not require formal coordination of care you may want to provide information in your waiting room or on your website. Remember to continually update the information in case cost of service, times or eligibility changes. This may include:

Boys and Girls Clubs

Food Pantries

Religious Supports

LGBTQIA+ Community Spaces and Clinics

Support Groups

You should document your coordination of care in an intervention plan as well as the date of referral. A copy of the Release of Information should also be placed in the client file.

Introducing the Process to the Client

The final phase of coordination of referrals involves the preparation and education of the client. The client needs to understand:

- Why the referral is necessary
- How the referral will provide support
- The process for utilizing the referral. (You can use all the information you gathered in your initial networking)

Clients often avoid reaching out to referrals due to fear of how they will be treated or not understanding the purpose or process. When we are able to describe the reasoning and process in detail, as well as answer questions and concerns, we increase the likelihood of the client's follow-through with the referral. This is especially important when client identities may have resulted in stigma, discrimination in previous service situations.

When referring clients for sexual health services I encourage you to be especially thoughtful about when you include the intervention in the treatment process. Gynecology and Urology doctors will inherently be invasive. Their expertise may be needed for symptoms related to dysfunction (erection difficulties, ejaculation difficulties, changes in dryness or lubrication). The referral will likely include an exam and blood draw.

For many of our clients they may have had medical trauma or mistreatment related to race, culture, legal status, gender, orientation, socio-economic status. We can ask our clients what previous experiences have been like. We can discuss their rights to fair, informed, and compassionate care. Acknowledging what has happened to them in the past and giving language about what they do deserve can be healing and empowering. It is helpful to practice examples of how they can advocate for themselves or end the service process when they do not feel cared for or respected. Giving clients tools and practice is good preparation. This is yet another space where we can model and help clients experience consent, giving permission and setting boundaries.

For many of our clients, the possibility of taking clothes off for an exam, being touched by a medical professional creates intense fear, panic, flashbacks. This is often the case when there is a history of sexual abuse. Letting your client know that the expertise may be necessary to relieve symptoms and we need to balance this with their need to feel safe. Pacing and preparation is truly necessary so as to not retraumatize an individual.

We can prepare clients for using referrals by walking through the process in the form of a guided visualization. The guided visualization in this form is a type of exposure therapy. The space of therapy allows the client to feel safe and to be able to pause and apply grounding techniques. By asking them to imagine themselves in the situation and describing the appointment step-by-step, we can create an exposure to the event. After each visualization exposure, ask how disturbing the event is from 0–10 scale to evaluate change. As disturbance decreases, we can also help install new skills within the visualization. New skills might include asking the doctor to describe what they are doing before they do it or asking the doctor to pause for a moment. Ask the client to imagine applying the new skill and then ask what they notice about their fear. The feeling of powerlessness often associated with medical exams can be changed by applying self-advocacy. It is not necessary for the exposure through visualization to result in a disturbance of zero before the client seeks care. Decreasing the disturbance, increasing sense of empowerment and skills for advocacy are important to evaluate readiness. The next section is a step-by-step guide to this process.

Guided Visualization for Medical Services

- Introduce the purpose of the exercise
- Ask the client to be aware of their position in the space where they are sitting.
- Call attention to areas of their body that may feel tense or uncomfortable.
- Encourage stretching out limbs or gently rotating neck to relieve tension in the body.
- Describe the process in as much detail as possible

Imagine you are entering the facility [insert name of specialist if possible]

There are people in the waiting room and they notice you as you enter. Notice how your body feels at this moment.

- Notice your breathing at this moment as you sit here in the room. If there is anxiety, you may notice some shallowness of breathing. Intentionally deepen and slow your breath.
- In your mind's eye, approach the reception area and provide your name [insert other material that may be needed such as insurance card].
- Imagine that your name is being called and you are escorted into the clinical room. There is a gown on the table and the medical assistant describes removing your clothing and getting dressed in the gown. The lighting is bright in the room, the walls are beige.
- Notice how your body feels as you imagine this. Are there questions you have to ask the medical assistant? Do you notice any concerns about safety coming up?
- Now you are waiting in the room with the medical gown on. There is a knock on the door and Dr. – enters. They have a white jacket on, a face mask. You notice their eyes are smiling and their voice sounds kind. They introduce themselves and you share your name. You are grateful the doctor has shared their pronouns. This experience feels different from past experiences at the doctor's office.
- The doctor refers to the referral completed by your therapist regarding –. They ask you to describe a bit of your history with this problem.
- Take a moment now to notice your breath and direct some long, deep, calming breaths into your gut. Practice in your head or aloud, asking the doctor for a moment to gather your thoughts. Remember that this is a place you have control and can make decisions.
- You ask the doctor to describe the – – (exam, procedure, etc.).
- The doctor describes the exam and shows you a diagram of what they will focus on during the exam.
- You ask about what it will feel like and if pain is common.
- The doctor assures you that you have complete control to stop the exam at any time. They share that they will be checking in with you verbally many times during the exam to see how you are feeling and ask if you need any support or to pause.
- Check in to see what emotions come to your mind as you imagine yourself in this process."
- Ask the client to center themselves back in the moment and open their eyes if this applies.
- As you take a moment to process the experience of this visualization focus on the techniques of breathing and noticing their body.
- Ask the client about the level of disturbance they are feeling at the end of the visualization. Ask the client to compare a past medical experience

with the visualization and notice differences. If at all possible, help them focus on differences in their own advocacy.

This visualization can be repeated to decrease disturbance, make slight changes, or expand on the visualization. Adding specific images such as pictures of the doctor or exam room, or even language of the treatment procedures, or pictures of tools used, can be additional help in exposure therapy element. As an example, I often ask clients to look at and even hold the dilators commonly used in treatment for genito-pelvic pain disorder.

In addition to the fear of being touched, the meaning associated with a referral can also be difficult for a client and important to explore. For a client seeking urology services related to concerns about Erectile Dysfunction, Delayed Ejaculation, shame may be associated with this intervention. The expectation that our bodies *should* function a certain way and are *failing*, or are not good enough, is commonly related to sexual difficulties. Media, social media, pornography, creates a false version of the human body as constantly hard, lubricated, thin, curvy, ready. . . . Sometimes clients want to address a problem that is not a medical problem, rather a problem of expectation or a problem of lack of education related to the human body. Just as we help our clients understand that sadness is an important emotion and often useful and we help them differentiate sadness from depression; we need to do the same important work related to sexual expectations of the body. Using the DOUPE assessment (described in Chapter 5) is a good way to understand how the problem is experienced and what the expectations are to resolve this problem. I often share with clients that:

Sex is ever-changing across the lifespan

Sex is always influenced by other life factors

Sex is often wonderful and always imperfect

Sex is variable from person to person and situation to situation.

We can help a client by discussing how age/time of life, stressors in other areas of life, expectations of self may be at the root of what they perceive is something wrong with them. Certainly, we do not need to deny a referral, but setting expectations for the referral, as well as opening the door to other considerations for interventions is important. Normalizing the experience of sexual difficulty goes a long way in decreasing shame, if it does exist.

In therapy we can assist clients in exploring what the appointment means about them, for them. Additional questions should include:

- How will you describe the problem you are experiencing?
- What are your expectations for the visit?
- What hope or goal to you have as the result of this treatment?
- Is there any type of intervention that will feel too fast or too invasive in this upcoming visit? (bloodwork, exam, testing)

Considerations Related to Gender Identity

As social workers and mental health workers, we work in advocacy and education to ensure safe and quality services for our clients. When creating a referral network there are many considerations related to safety for gender non-binary, questioning, and transgender clients. Some questions that should always be asked of an individual or agency you would like to add to your referral network:

- Does your intake paperwork include chosen name and pronouns?
- Is staff trained to use chosen name/pronouns?
- Is there staff training related to care for gender non-binary and transgender clients?
- Are there gender-inclusive restrooms?
- Are staff informed of inclusive medical care for gender non-binary and transgender clients?
- Do you have a history of successful work with this community?
- Why is working with this community important to you?

We can increase the likelihood of clients utilizing referrals if we share with our clients what to expect in terms of gender safety and gender-informed care. As social workers this is imperative work related to our principle of social justice.

Beyond Medical and Social Services

Our field is changing to respond to a need for integration of mind, body, and spirit, as well as integration of formal and informal supports. Doing thorough work in identifying your network of referrals and providing organized and informative coordination of services ensures you can provide a meaningful treatment approach and focus your skills on your specific areas of expertise. Many of our clients will want to explore solutions outside of traditional social and medical support. While these treatments and solutions may not be evidence-based and may be outside the scope of our formal process, we can still play a role in helping clients navigate resources, understand their treatment goals and approach the process as an advocate for themselves. These resources may include:

Religious instituations

Spiritual retreats

Holistic medicine

Massage therapy

Energy work

Breath work

Sexual surrogacy

Martial arts

Pet therapy

As mental health professionals we hold a careful balance in not providing formal referrals or speaking outside of our area of practice while remaining open and supportive to areas clients may want to explore. We can ask some of the same questions we used to introduce the process of a formal referral:

- Why is the service/expert necessary?
- How will it provide support/change?

We can also help the client to think about how to advocate for themselves while seeking this additional service. One of the reasons this is important is because they have identified the service related to a presenting problem or related to an intervention and we are assisting them with in the mental health domain. A couple examples include:

A client seeking services related to Prolonged Grief Disorder hopes that massage and energy work may offer some relief to how disconnected she feels from herself and her body.

Or

An adolescent who has been in therapy to address Major Depressive Disorder will be moving away to attend college. They want to explore pet therapy as a way to manage depressive symptoms.

Or

A client is in treatment for Gender Dysphoria and would like to explore dancing and music as a way to feel more connected to their body.

Navigating these resources with clients requires us to lead with naming our area of expertise and what is outside of that expertise.

"As a mental health clinician my expertise is related to evidence-based treatments for your diagnosis."

We can then honor the client's interest in exploring the specific resource as a way of intervening with symptoms.

"It is inspiring and hopeful that you want to add some new resources to improving your well-being and quality of life."

Then we can help the client think about ways to find quality resources in the area of service. We may know some word-of-mouth referrals, online groups as well as thinking about specific concerns the client should consider.

Are experts in this resource area licensed or credentialed by any governing body?

What is some of the specific language used in this field?

What is average cost of the service?

Are there health or safety concerns associated with the service?

When clients step outside of their comfort zone, they will be more likely to feel successful using the service if we can help them in preparation. We can also increase safety by helping clients think through the specifics of new services. These brave, new experiences often help clients develop increased confidence and independence and expand the resources they rely on to care for themselves. Our support, enthusiasm, and advocacy are a big part of the joining element of the collaborative relationship.

Mental health professionals often underestimate the importance of quality coordination of care in treatment planning. Often professionals are dismissive of this work because it feels more like case management than clinical treatment planning. My hope is that this chapter allows the reader to consider the details that can be introduced to referrals and coordination of care. Dedicated planning to building a quality network will allow you to focus your time and skills within your expertise while ensuring clients are able to address a diversity of needs associated with the presenting problem.

Questions for Reflection and Discussion

When considering the community you practice in, what are the agencies that support sexual health? Is there access to the uninsured, undocumented, LGBTQI+ community and disabled community?

What sexual health services are most needed in your community?

The Road Forward   **15**

Introduction

Social workers, psychologists, counselors, and therapists, as well as doctors, physician's assistants, and nurse practitioners are busy all over the world addressing issues of sexuality, sexual health, and intimacy. During the time you took to read this book, a social worker sat on the porch during a home visit. He guided a mother and teenager through a difficult conversation about gender identity and sexuality. A doctor patiently discussed vaginal pain and difficult sex with a patient before a gynecological exam. A nurse distributed internal and external condoms and lubrication packets while discussing safety and pleasure basics regarding anal sex. This work is not often described as the work of heroes, but it is.

As discussed throughout this book, acknowledgement, and validation of sexuality needs to be a core component of ethical mental health practice. It can feel complicated to consider what to discuss and how to discuss it in the diversity of practice spaces within which mental health professionals work. The way that we do our work is to encourage, validate, analyze, challenge, resource, educate, and advocate. The areas we address are health, relationships, safety, regulation, security, attachment, stabilization. There may be a lot of learning curves in the work, but we can prepare for a baseline of sexual health education and resourcing to begin the work.

DOI: 10.4324/9781003166382-16

Resources

Sex toys are an important way for individuals to get to know their bodies as well as adding to their experience of intimacy. In my years as an educator and therapist, I have learned that people have a great variance in terms of information and comfort with sex toys. Here is some basic information about sex devices and tips in safety and purpose.

Vibrators/dildos: Dildos are often made to mimic the appearance of a penis. They are most often used to insert into a vagina or anus. Vibrators come in various shapes, including mimicking the look of a penis. Some vibrators are shaped to focus on the g-spot, an internal spot of the vagina that can be associated with increased pleasure or orgasm. For many, there is a preference for a long shape that does not mimic the look of a penis. Increasing marketing highlights ergonomically-sculpting to please all body types. There is more flexibility about how these toys could be used and they do not resemble a penis. For instance, the bullet is a vibrator that can be used on various body parts. The we-vibe is a circular vibrator with a slight opening to allow for inserting. It could be used for vaginal, clitoral or anal pleasure. This can be explored solo or partnered. The advances in marketing that includes shapes, colors, and flexibility, makes these toys more approachable for a diversity of bodies, genders, and sexual expression.

> **Clitoral vibrators**: Some vibrators focus only externally. This may include an egg-shaped vibrator that can pulse on top of the clitoris or other toys that provide a suction sensation. It is more common for individuals to experience clitoral orgasm than vaginal orgasm. However, for some, the sensitivity of the clitoris can make direct contact painful.

> **Constriction rings (aka cock rings)**: These are placed at the shaft of the penis to reduce blood flow away from the penis. They can be used as an aid for individuals with erectile dysfunction. The vibrating versions also are used in partnered sexual experience to increase pleasure in clitoral or anal stimulation.

> **Flesh lights**: The flesh light looks externally like an over-sized flashlight. The internal chamber replicates the texture of a vagina, anus or oral surface. Flesh lights allow someone with a penis to masturbate into the flesh light and experience a similar feeling to penetration. Flesh lights can assist individuals with premature ejaculation in exposure to the sensation.

Anal plugs: Anal plugs or butt plugs are teardrop-shaped with a base. The base is very important so that the plug does not get pulled into the anus and become difficult to retrieve. Some may experience prostate orgasm through anal play. Intensified orgasms are also common when pairing anal play with other forms of sexual arousal. Some prefer to stick with anal plugs and others may use plugs to orient themselves with anal play and move on to inserting dildos, vibrators, vibrating beads, or wands.

As mental health professionals it is helpful to be informed about sex toys so we can be familiar with different ways individuals may explore intimacy. We can also encourage individuals to educate themselves about the use of sex toys to increase information about pleasure, self-exploration or building sexual confidence. In Chapter 11, the PLISSIT model was described that teaches us to intervene with the least invasive techniques possible. Sometimes experimentation with sex toys can be a simple suggestion that resolve concerns for clients.

Consider this brief interaction with a client that might include conversation about sex toys:

Client Anna has been seeing her social worker for about a month. She is focused on addressing symptoms of generalized anxiety disorder. She shared in this meeting with her social worker that she really likes her girlfriend but she is so overwhelmed with the idea of being intimate that she sometimes thinks it would be better to just break up.

Social Worker (SW):	Anna, you've talked a lot about how much you enjoy spending time with your girlfriend. It seems like ending the relationship would be really sad for you. I wonder if we could come up with solutions that are in between breaking up and all the worry and anxiety that you are facing now?
Anna:	You are right. I really like Viv so much. It's not so much that she pressures me. It's just that she wants to be sexual after many months of dating. I keep putting it off because I don't really know what I'm doing.
SW:	When you say you don't know what you are doing, does that mean you don't know what you like or what Viv enjoys sexually?
Anna:	Oh, Viv is really confident. She has already told me lots of things she would like to do and she has told me what turns her on. That's what is intimidating! I don't know

	what to tell her about me. It is so intimidating and gives me so much anxiety.
SW:	It might be a lot less intimidating if you let yourself figure this out on your own terms first. Have you ever masturbated?
Anna:	I try but I don't think I totally get it. I mean it feels pretty good but I don't get to the place that most people talk about. I have never had an orgasm.
SW:	I wonder if it might be helpful to get a sex toy that would allow you to explore a bit more.
Anna:	I feel sort of repulsed by those giant pink dicks they sell at those sex stores.
SW:	Oh, I get what you are saying. The cool thing is there is actually a lot of different types of toys or devices you can buy now that don't look anything like a penis. Some of them are only a few inches long. Those are called bullets. There are others that just look like an egg and you could use them just externally. They just vibrate.
Anna:	Oh, I didn't realize that.
SW:	You can even order them online.
Anna:	I could try that.
SW:	Maybe get started just getting to know your own body and this might help you gain confidence in talking to Viv about what you like.

The issue of anxiety and relationship lead the social worker and Anna into a conversation about intimacy and sex toys. Helping Anna find ways to explore her own body will hopefully increase knowledge and confidence, thus reducing some of the anxiety she is experiencing in her relationship. When we discuss sex toys, we should also share some basic tips on hygiene and safety.

- When purchasing sex toys, it will tell you if they can be placed in water. Some can even be submerged. Many individuals feel most comfortable or have privacy when in the shower or bath, so this is helpful information.
- Toys used for any type of penetration should always be used with lubrication. Water or silicone-based lubricants are safe to use with toys, but oil-based lubricants can often be harmful for toys.
- Washing toys is important and should be done after every use. Soap and water can be used and spray on cleaners are also available when you purchase toys.

- Toys for vaginal insertion and anal insertion should be separated so as to not cause contamination that can easily lead to urinary tract infections.
- Anal toys should always have a base that stays on the outside of the body and allows the object to be pulled out when exploration is done.

This could be expanded in the conversation with Anna:

SW: When you go online to purchase a toy you may want to also buy some lubrication and toy cleaner. If you keep these in a safe place next to your toy, you have everything you need to make it safe, healthy, and accessible.

Anna: Do you think I'll need lubricant? I thought that was just in case you weren't into it and needed some extra.

SW: Everyone's body lubricates at different amounts and that even fluctuates at different times in a person's cycle and can be influenced by mood. Lubrication also increases with arousal. When you are beginning masturbating your body may not have much lubrication so having some on hand to place on the toy or on your body can be very helpful. It will make it more enjoyable and helps to take care of the delicate tissue.

Anna: Good information.

SW: I always remind people to go to the bathroom afterwards. Urinating helps clean out any bacteria from the body. Then you can clean off the toy and you are all set.

Like information about medication, we can help ensure that individuals use sex toys properly and safely if we walk them through the process.

Sex Aids and Disability

As discussed in Chapter 8, disabled individuals are often viewed as being without sexual desire or a sexuality. Conversations about sexual health and access to privacy or ways to be sexual is often kept from disabled individuals. Caregivers and family members may feel uncomfortable discussing the topic or ensuring there is an opportunity to be sexual. Mental health professionals often play an important role of acknowledging the individual's sexual self, connecting them to resources and advocating for their access and privacy.

Rodney was 30 years old when he met with a social worker at a veteran's program. The social worker discussed employment, education, and training interests. They also explored support systems. They completed an assessment related to mood, anxiety, and trauma symptoms. Rodney was in a wheelchair and had learned one year ago that he would likely never walk. He returned from war in Afghanistan to his wife and their five-year-old child. He felt grateful to be alive but expressed that finding his way in his new identity was overwhelming. Asking about his sexual health and intimacy made a big difference to Rodney.

Social Worker (SW):	Rodney, I've asked you a lot of questions about your health and well-being and I'd like to include questions about your sexual health and intimacy.
Rodney:	Well, that's refreshing. No one ever asks about that and it sure is hard to figure things out in that department.
SW:	Can you tell me a little bit more about what's been hard to figure out?
Rodney:	Well, I can still get it up but trying to figure out how to do things now that my legs don't work is really kind of difficult. I think it's hard for my wife too. I know she wants to be close but we haven't figured out how to actually do it or make things sexy since I came home. [He starts to cry and lowers his head.] I miss her so much and I worry that we will never find our way.
SW:	I am so glad to hear that there is a desire there for you. So much has changed and you and your wife deserve support in figuring out this new terrain of your sex life together. It sounds like you and your wife haven't had a chance to talk about this much?
Rodney:	Yep, I don't really know how to bring it up. Sometimes she will reach out and touch me at night or even give me a blow job. That's amazing but I want to have sex.
SW:	So, having penetrative sex is something really important for you and maybe your wife too?
Rodney:	Yep, I used to always be on top. When I think about it, I think we can find ways to do it now, but it might take some figuring.
SW:	A lot of the veterans I've worked with have benefited from having some simple props that help them position

	in different ways. It might be useful to take a look at some websites that sell the aids and even have photographs demonstrating the different positions. We can look at them here and maybe think about some ways to raise the topic with your wife.
Rodney:	That sounds like a great place to start!

Several companies sell devices that are firm cushions that help with positioning. Wedges and ramps serve to help couples position themselves to enable sexual experiences or new sexual experiences. Demonstrated in the brief client/social worker transcript is the importance of recognizing intimacy as a part of the individual's well-being. This is the biggest error of mental health professionals and all other professionals working with individuals with disabilities. It is perhaps most important with this population to raise the topic because it may be the only conversation that can lead to vital access to resources that allow for sexual experiences.

Technology is elevating the possibility of sexual experiences for individuals who are severely limited in movement. Designers are creating full-body suits that allow individuals to access multiple sensations of hearing, smell, and touch. Assistance is limited to the individual receiving assistance putting the suit on.

Other devices exist that offer assistance in masturbation. This is an interactive masturbator that is hands-free. It requires the assistance of placing the device on the penis. Advocacy with caregivers or family members surrounding the importance of sexual experiences and privacy may be necessary.

Finding new ways to experience stimulation and pleasure is often explored through kink. It is a common pathway for individuals with chronic pain as well as disability to explore new ways to experience sexuality. When there are barriers to the common way of being sexual, often penetrative sex, individuals reach out for information on other ways to experience pleasure. Clients may express interest in exploration of kink or may have a partner who is interested. As mental health professionals we can help individuals consider what they want to experience as well as why they want to experience it. Navigating these questions will help an individual think more specifically about what they are trying to achieve. We also want to help individuals by educating about and identifying boundaries, limits, and safe words.

Consider Kayla's conversation with a social worker at a community mental health setting. Kayla was 19 years old. She had been seeing her social worker for approximately six weeks. She had experienced sexual trauma in the last year and was seeking help in addressing the trauma and dating again. She came into a session and shared with her social worker that she was going to "open up more" with the new guy she was dating. She said he was "kind of kinky" and she was excited to explore this.

Social Worker (SW):	I'm glad to see you excited and considering new things that might be pleasurable. Tell me a little bit more about what you would like to explore.
Kayla:	Um, I don't know, just like spanking or some handcuffs or something.
SW:	Sure. All of that could be a part of something pleasurable. Can we think more specifically about what is exciting to you?
Kayla:	I mean sure, I guess.
SW:	If we think about bondage, being a form of restraint or restraining someone else, do you think you would like that?
Kayla:	Maybe, but it might make me a little nervous because of my sexual assault. It could be fun to restrain my partner though.
SW:	Okay, so that might be interesting or possibly pleasurable. You might like to explore that. What about the idea of dominance or submission, meaning either being in charge or being the one who is taken charge of. Does that sound pleasurable, interesting, or maybe even unsafe?
Kayla:	Well, it is interesting. I'm realizing if we were to do this and I was the one being dominated, I would want to make sure I could stop when I needed to.
SW:	That is so great that you are aware of that. Actually, that is the best practice of people who are kinky. They use a safe word that is totally unrelated to the sex stuff. That way, when the word is said, it sticks out and is clear. You might say, "no" or "stop" as part of the sexy scene and your partner wouldn't know you weren't just being in the moment.
Kayla:	Oh, so I would use a random word like. . . pickle.
SW:	Exactly! The other thing you can consider is if you think you might want to explore pain in some form.

Kayla:	Maybe, but it isn't where I want to start.
SW:	That's good. That is your limit for the time being. It is important to express that to your partner. You also want to think about what your boundary is in restraint or restraining or dominating. Maybe you could think about those two questions on your own first and then talk to your partner about them.
Kayla:	What are they again?
SW:	What do you want to experience? Why do you want to experience it?

Throughout this book we have discovered ways to embrace an individual's sexual expression. Individuals are best suited to explore when we help them think about ways to be physically and emotionally safe in their experiences. Referrals and information are important for individuals to be safely sexual:

- Regular exams that include STD and HIV testing
- Information and access to inexpensive or free contraception
- Information and access to PEP (post-exposure prophylaxis) is for possible exposure to HIV to prevent the virus from invading your body. PEP must be taken within 72 hours of exposure to the virus.
- Information and access to PREP (Pre-exposure prophylaxis) is taken on a regular basis to prevent getting HIV. It is 99% effective when taken as prescribed.
- Access to and education to use vaginal condoms, dental dams and lubrication.

As mental health professionals our basic sexual health education and advocacy should acknowledge every human's sexual self, provide access to privacy, resources, and access to safety and well-being and education about how to use resources responsibly. In the case of individuals that are dependent due to age or need for care, we must also serve in a role of advocacy.

Conclusion

The introduction of this book shared the stories of Betty, Angel, and Cortez. Sometimes I can't help but rewind their stories in my mind and consider how things might have been different if they had access to education about their bodies and space to explore issues of pleasure, sexuality, and consent. The thread of sexual trauma that was at the root of all their stories may have been addressed earlier. Maybe behavior wouldn't have become so out of control, maybe the numbing, sexual violence and AIDS wouldn't have been the outcome. Rewinding the story is painful because I can't go back in time. It is important to keep their memories with me because they inspire me to intervene at all the right moments that are occurring now. Talking about sex can change the world. Thousands are making this happen right now.

Checking in With Case Study: Following Up With Roseanna

We met Roseanna at the beginning of the book. She had worked hard to access services, even making up some information in the intake, to get in the door. Roseanna spoke confidently that sex work was not the problem or a trauma; anorgasmia in her personal relationship was her focus. I leaned into her expertise about her work. I asked her how she managed boundaries and consent in her work. Roseanna had been mentored by a group of loving and supportive people when she started as a sex worker. They had talked about safety and negotiation openly. Roseanna acknowledged that there had been some scary incidents in her work over the years, but she handled them well and gained confidence in herself.

When Roseanna talked about her relationship with her partner, she reflected on a loving relationship with a patient man. We used some of the interventions that have been discussed in this book to explore the biological, emotional, and relationship underpinnings of sexual experiences. Roseanna had a lot of information about her body and what felt pleasurable. She described a feeling of desire and arousal but couldn't quite "fully let go." When I explored that language with her, Roseanna became very thoughtful and curious. She realized that she was "a little too good at being in charge." Her partner was thoughtful and gentle but rarely dominant or "in charge." Roseanna wondered if it would help her fully "let go," if she felt less in charge.

We used the intervention of sexual scripts. Roseanna shared some of her fantasies and realized that she had some interest in exploring bondage and dominance/submission play in her sexual relationship with her partner. She expressed hesitance in communicating this with her partner. Through journaling on her own and roleplaying in session, Roseanna was able to identify her fears and felt more prepared to discuss her sexual needs with her partner. Roseanna reported that her partner was really interested in incorporating BDSM practices into their relationship. I recommended a book that served as a wonderful introduction into BDSM.

Evaluating the goals of treatment, success was not just based on achieving orgasm, but the increased insight into her sexual needs and the increased communication about sexual expression with her partner. For the record, Roseanna did eventually have an orgasm. She and her partner discovered so much about themselves and their relationship by opening a new door into intimacy through BDSM. Listening to Roseanna's expertise about her goals for therapy was imperative to success in our therapeutic work. It was necessary to understand that anorgasmia, or female orgasmic disorder, as identified in the DSM-5-TR, had biological, psychological, and relational underpinnings. It was also important to understand why an orgasm felt important to Roseanna. I would have addressed treatment much differently if her need for an orgasm was about a performance failure. I would likely have focused on interventions to explore and evaluate pleasure differently using the body map or mindful touch.

Roseanna's case reminds us that every case is unique. Roseanna had terrific insight about her body, so psychoeducation about masturbation or lubrication wasn't as important. Even though many mental health professionals had assumed trauma was the source of her problem, their beliefs were related to a stigma about sex work. Trauma processing was not a core part of Roseanna's treatment needs. Helping her listen to her language and honor her sexual needs was so important. When Roseanna was able to give herself permission to desire being dominated in sexual experiences with her partner, she was then able to communicate that with confidence.

When students are poised to graduate the most common fear they express is "what if I don't know what to say?" I think that is less about being embarrassed and more about a fear about being unable to help the client. The theory of our work is our foundation. When we consider being a professional in a room with a client we wonder, what does this look like in practice? I have based every assessment and intervention in a case study and step-by-step guides. These are the tools to incorporate sex therapy practices in your work. You will gain confidence through using them and perfect your comfort and engagement with the tools over time. The biggest error, perhaps the only error, is not opening the conversation.

Good luck! This is the work of heroes. Talking about sex will change the world.

Questions for Reflection and Discussion

What do you hope to use from this text as you move forward in your career?

References

American Association of Sex Educators, Counselors, and Therapists. (2022). *Sex therapy certification guidelines*. Retrieved from aasect.org.

American Psychiatric Association. (2022). *Diagnostic and statistical manual of mental disorders* (5th Edition Tr).

Behrens, K. G. (2020). A principled ethical approach to intersex pediatric surgeries. *BMC Medical Ethics, 21*. https://doi-org.proxy.lib.umich.edu/10.1186/s12910-020-00550-x.

Bennecke, E., Bernstein, S., Lee, P., van de Grift, T. C., Nordenskjöld, A., Rapp, M., Simmonds, M., Streuli, J. C., Thyen, U., & Wiesemann, C. (2021). Early genital surgery in disorders/differences of sex development: Patients' perspectives. *Archives of Sexual Behavior, 50*(3), 913–923. https://doi-org.proxy.lib.umich.edu/10.1007/s10508-021-01953-6.

Betchen, S. J. (2003). Suggestions for improving intimacy in couples in which one partner has attention-deficit/hyperactivity disorder. *Journal of Sex & Marital Therapy, 29*, 103–124.

Bigler, M. O. (2005). Harm reduction as a practice and prevention model for social work. *Journal of Baccalaureate Social Work, 10*(2), 69–86. https://doiorg.proxy.lib.umich.edu/10.18084/1084-7219.10.2.69.

Bigras, N., et al. (2017). Cumulative adverse childhood experiences and sexual satisfaction in sex therapy patients: What role for symptom complexity. *Journal of Sexual Medicine, 14*, 444–454. http://dx.doi.org/10.1016/j.jsxm.2017.01.013.

Braun-Harvey, D., & Vigorito, M. (2016). *Treating out of control sexual behavior: Rethinking sex addiction*. Springer Publishing Company.

Brown, S. L., Seymour, N. E., Mitchell, S. M., et al. (2022). Interpersonal risk factors, sexual, and gender minority status, and suicidal ideation: Is BDSM disclosure protective? *Archives of Sexual Behavior, 51*, 1091–1101. https://doi-org.proxy.lib.umich.edu/10.1007/s10508-021-02186-3.

Burke-Harris, N. (2018). *The deepest well: Healing the long-term effects of childhood adversity*. HarperCollins Publisher.

Burns, T., et al. (2017). Graduate counseling psychology training in sex and sexuality: An exploratory analysis. *The Counseling Psychologist, 45*(4), 504–527. doi:10.1177/001100001771465.

Carnes, P. (2001). *Out of the shadows: Understanding sexual addiction.* Hazelden Publishing.

Castellini, G., Lelli, L., Lo Sauro, C., Fioravani, G., Vignozzi, L., Maggi, M., . . . Ricca, V. (2012). Anorectic and bulimic patients suffer from relevant sexual dysfunctions. *The Journal of Sexual Medicine, 9*(10), 2590–2599.

Cavanaugh, T. (2019). *Sexual health history: Talking sex with gender non-conforming and trans patients* [Advancing Excellence in Transgender Health]. Fenway Health.

Coleman, E. (2002, February). Promoting sexual health and responsible sexual behavior: An introduction. *Journal of Sex Research, 39*(1), 3–6. doi:10.1080/00224490209552111.

Coleman, E., Bockting, W., Botzer, M., Cohen-Kettenis, P., DeCuypere, G., Feldman, J., Fraser, L., Green, J., Knudson, G., Meyer, W. J., Monstrey, S., Adler, R. K., Brown, G. R., Devor, A. H., Ehrbar, R., Ettner, R., Eyler, E., Garofalo, R., Karasic, D. H., . . . Zucker, K. (2012). Standards of care for the health of transsexual, transgender, and gender-nonconforming people, version 7. *International Journal of Transgenderism, 13*(4), 165–232. https://doi.org/10.1080/15532739.2011.700873.

Dana, D. (2020). *Polyvagal flip chart: Understanding the science of safety.* W.W. Norton & Company.

Diamond, L. (2008). *Sexual fluidity: Understanding women's love and desire.* Harvard University Press.

Driscoll, C., & Flanagan, E. (2016). Sexual problems and posttraumatic stress disorder following sexual trauma: A meta-analytic review. *Psychology and Psychotherapy: Theory, Research, and Practice, 89,* 351–367. doi:10.111/papt.12077.

Drucker, D. (2010). Male sexuality and Alfred Kinsey's 0–6 scale: Toward "A sound understanding of the realities of sex". *Journal of Homosexuality, 57,* 1105–1123. doi:10.1080/00918369.2010.508314.

Florence, A. (2019). Gatekeeping hormone replacement therapy for transgender patients is dehumanizing. *Journal of Medical Ethics, 45*(7), 480. http://dx.doi.org.proxy.lib.umich.edu/10.1136/medethics-2018-105293.

Foley, S. (2015). Biopsychosocial assessment and treatment of sexual problems in older age. *Current Sexual Health, 7,* 80–88. doi:10.1007/s11930-015-0047-9.

Foley, S., Kope, S., & Sugrue, D. (2012). *Sex matters for women: A complete guide to taking care of your sexual self.* The Guilford Press.

Follette, V. M., Briere, J., Rozelle, D., Hopper, J. W., & Rome, D. I. (Eds.). (2014). *Mindfulness-oriented interventions for trauma: Integrating contemplative practices.* Guilford Publications.

Fontanesi, L., et al. (2021). Hypersexuality and trauma: A mediation and moderation model from psychopathology to problematic sexual behavior. *Journal of Affective Disorders, 281,* 631–637. https://doi.org/10.1016/j.jad.2020.11.100.

Freek, P. W., et al. (2021). Patient-reported outcomes after genital gender-affirming surgery with versus without urethral lengthening in transgender men. *Journal of Sexual Medicine, 18*(5), 974–981. https://doi-org.proxy.lib.umich.edu/10.1016/j.jsxm.2021.03.002.

García-Blanco, A., García-Portilla, M. P., Fuente-Tomás, L. de la, Batalla, M., Sánchez-Autet, M., Arranz, B., Safont, G., Arqués, S., Livianos, L., & Sierra, P. (2020). Sexual dysfunction and mood stabilizers in long-term stable patients with bipolar disorder. *Journal of Sexual Medicine, 17*(5), 930–940. https://doi-org.proxy.lib.umich.edu/10.1016/j.jsxm.2020.01.032.

Ghadigaonkar, D., & Murthy, P. (2019). Sexual dysfunction in persons with substance use disorders. *Journal of Psychosexual Health, 1*(2), 117–121. doi:10.1177/2631831819849365.

Ghosh, A., Kathiravan, S., Sharma, K., & Mattoo, S. K. (2022). A scoping review of the prevalence and correlates of sexual dysfunction in adults with substance use disorders. *Journal of Sexual Medicine, 19*(2), 216–233. https://doiorg.proxy.lib.umich.edu/10.1016/j.jsxm.2021.11.018.

Gitlin, M. J. (1994). Psychotropic medications and their effects on sexual function: Diagnosis, biology, and treatment approaches. *Journal of Clinical Psychiatry, 9,* 406–413.

Gordon, E. (2020). A medical education recommendation for improving sexual health and humanism and professionalism. *Sexual Medicine Review,* 1–13. https://doi.org/10.1016/j.sxmr.2020.10.002.

Gordon, W. M. (2002). Sexual obsessions and obsessive-compulsive disorder. *Sexual and Relationship Therapy, 17*(4), 343–354.

Green, E. R., & Maurer, L. M. (2015). The teaching transgender toolkit: A facilitator's guide to increasing knowledge, decreasing prejudice & building skills. *Planned Parenthood of the Southern Finger Lakes: Out for Health.* ISBN: 978-0-9966783-0-8.

Hansen-Brown, A. A., & Jefferson, S. E. (2022). Perceptions of and stigma toward bdsm practitioners. *Current Psychology: A Journal for Diverse Perspectives on Diverse Psychological Issues.* https://doi-org.proxy.lib.umich.edu/10.1007/s12144-022-03112-z.

Harris, M. S. F.-B., Goodrum, B. A. F.-B., & Krempasky, C. N. F.-B. W.-B. (2022). An introduction to gender-affirming hormone therapy for transgender and gender-nonbinary patients. *Nurse Practitioner, 47*(3), 18–28. https://doi-org.proxy.lib.umich.edu/10.1097/01.NPR.0000819612.24729.c7.

Henrich, R., & Trawinski, C. (2016). Social and therapeutic challenges facing polyamorous clients. *Sexual and Relationships Therapy, 31*(3), 376–390. https://doi.org/10.1080/1468 1994.2016.1174331.

Herbenick, D. (2018). Women's experience with genital touching, sexual pleasure, and orgasm: Results from a U.S. probability sample of women ages 18–94. *Journal of Sex and Marital Therapy, 44*(2), 201–212. https://doi.org/10.1080/0092623x.2017.1346530.

Herman, J. (1995). *Trauma and recover: The aftermath of violence–from domestic violence to political terror.* Basic Books.

Hoffman, D. (2017). *You and your gender identity: A guide to discovery.* Skyhorse Publishing.

Hogben, M., et al. (2015). A systemic review of sexual health interventions for adults: Narrative evidence. *Journal of Sex Research, 52*(4), 444–469. doi:10.1080/00224499.201 4.973100.

Johnson, S. (2019). *Attachment theory in practice: Emotionally focused therapy (EFT) with individuals, couples, and families.* Guilford Press.

Kendurkar, A., & Brinder, K. (2008). Major depressive disorder, obsessive-compulsive disorder, and generalized anxiety disorder: Do the sexual dysfunctions differ? *Primary Care Companion to the Journal of Clinical Psychiatry, 10,* 299–305.

Kennedy. (2013, August 9). *Mira Bellweather and "fucking trans women" zine: The Autostraddle interview.* Retrieved from www.autostraddle.com/mira-bellwether-author-and-illustrator-of-fucking-trans-women-zine-the-autostraddle-interview/.

Kraus, S., et al. (2018). Compulsive sexual behavior disorder in the ICD-11. *World Psychiatry, 17,* 1.

Kubota, S., & Nakazawa, E. (2022). Concept and implications of sexual consent for education: A systematic review of empirical studies. *Sexual and Relationship Therapy*. https://doi-org.proxy.lib.umich.edu/10.1080/14681994.2022.2039617.

Kumsar, N. A., Kumsar, Ş., & Dilbaz, N. (2016). Sexual dysfunction in men diagnosed as substance use disorder. *Andrologia*, 48(10), 1229–1235. https://doi-org.proxy.lib.umich.edu/10.1111/and.12566.

Ladson, D., & Welton, R. (2007). Recognizing and managing erotic and eroticized transferences. *Psychiatry*, 4(4), 47–50.

Levin, R. J. (2008). Critically revisiting aspects of the human sexual response cycle of Masters and Johnson: Correcting errors and suggesting modifications. *Sexual and Relationship Therapy*, 23(4), 393–399. https://doi-org.proxy.lib.umich.edu/10.1080/14681990802488816.

Levine, P. (1999). *Healing trauma: A pioneering program for restoring the wisdom of the body*. Sounds True, Inc.

Ling, T. J., Geiger, C. J., Hauck, J. M., et al. (2022). BDSM, non-monogamy, consent, and stigma navigation: Narrative experiences. *Archives of Sexual Behavior*, 51, 1075–1089. https://doi-org.proxy.lib.umich.edu/10.1007/s10508-021-02191-6.

Linschoten, M., Weiner, L., & Avery-Clark, C. (2016). Sensate focus: A critical literature review. *Sexual and Relational Therapy*, 31(2). http://dx.doi.org/10.1080/14681994.2015.1127909.

McClelland, S. (2010). Intimate justice: A critical analysis of sexual satisfaction. *Social and Personality Psychology Compass*, 4(9), 663–680. doi:10.111/j175-9004.2010.00293x.

Miller, W., & Rollnick, S. (2013). *Motivational interviewing: Helping people change*. Guilford Press.

Morin, J. (1995). *The erotic mind: Unlocking the inner sources of sexual passion and fulfillment*. HarperCollins Publishers.

Nagoski, E. (2015). *Come as you are: The surprising new science that will transform your sex life*. Simon and Schuster.

New, C. M., Batchelor, L. C., Schimmel-Bristow, A., Schaeffer-Smith, M., Magsam, E., Bridges, S. K., Brown, E. L., & McKenzie, T. (2021). In their own words: Getting it right for kink clients. *Sexual and Relationship Therapy*. doi:10.1080/14681994.2021.1965112.

Ogden, P. (2006). *Trauma and the body: A sensorimotor approach to psychotherapy*. W.W. Norton and Company.

Orenstein, P. (2016). *What young women believe about their own sexual pleasure* [Video]. Ted Conferences.

Perleman, R. (2012). Helen Singer Kaplan's legacy and the future of sexual medicine. *Journal of Sexual Medicine*, 9, 138.

Peterson, F, Bley, J., & Frobotta, F. (2016). *The gender revolution & new sexual health: Celebrating unlimited diversity of the human sexual hypercube*. Routledge.

Pleak, R. R. (2011). Gender identity issues in youth: Opportunities, terminologies, histories, and advancements. *Child and Adolescent Psychiatric Clinics of North America*, 20(4), 601–625. https://doi-org.proxy.lib.umich.edu/10.1016/j.chc.2011.08.006.

Pulverman, C., & Meston, C. (2019). Sexual dysfunction in women with a history of childhood sexual abuse: The role of sexual shame. *Psychological Trauma: Theory, Research, Practice, and Policy*, 12(3), 299. https://doi.org/10.1037/tra0000506.

Quinn, C., Happell, B., & Browne, G. (2011). Sexuality and consumers of mental health services: The impact of gender and boundary issues. *Issues Mental Health Nursing*, 32(3), 170–176. doi:10.3109/01612840.2010.531518.

Rancourt, K., et al. (2015). Talking about sex when sex is painful: Dyadic sexual communication is associated with women's pain, and couples' sexual and psychological outcomes in provoked vestibuludynia. *Archives of Sexual Behavior, 45,* 1933–1944. doi:10.1007/s10508-015-0670-6.

Ratner, E. S., et al. (2011). Sexual satisfaction in the elderly female population: A special focus on women with gynecologic pathology. *Maturitas, 70*(3), 210–215. doi:10.1016/j. maturitas.2011.07.015.

Reed, G. M., et al. (2016). Disorders related to sexuality and gender identity in the ICD-11: Revising the ICD-10 classification based on current scientific evidence, best clinical practices, and human rights considerations. *World Psychiatry, 15*(3), 205–221. doi:10.1002/wps.20354.

Reise, S. P., & Wright, T. M. (1996). Personality traits, cluster B personality disorders, and sociosexuality. *Journal of Research in Personality, 30*(1), 128–136.

Salomaa, A. C., Livingston, N. A., Bryant, W. T., Herbitter, C., Harper, K., Sloan, C. A., Hinds, Z., Gyuro, L., Valentine, S. E., & Shipherd, J. C. (2022). A bottom-up approach to developing a unified trauma-minority stress model for transgender and gender diverse people. *Psychological Trauma: Theory, Research, Practice, and Policy.* https://doi-org.proxy.lib.umich.edu/10.1037/tra0001373.supp (Supplemental)

Schwartz, R., & Sweezy, M. (2020). *Internal family systems* (2nd Edition). Guilford Press.

Sexuality Information and Education Council of the United States. (2004). *Guidelines for comprehensive sexuality education: Kindergarten-12th grade* (3rd Edition). SIECUS.

Shapiro, F. (2017). *Eye movement desensitization reprocessing: Basic principles, protocols, and procedures.* Guildford Press.

Siegal, D. (2010). *The mindful therapist: A clinician's guide to mindset and neural integration.* W.W. Norton & Company.

Siegal, D., & Hartzell, M. (2003). *Parenting from the inside out: How a deeper self-understanding can help you raise children who thrive.* The Penguin Group.

Sokolowski, M. (2012). Sex, Dementia, and the Nursing Home: Ethical Issues of Reflection. *Journal of Ethics in Mental Health, 7*(1).

Southall, D. J. L., & Combes, H. A. (2020). Clinical psychologists' views about talking to people with psychosis about sexuality and intimacy: A q-methodological study. *Sexual and Relationship Therapy.* doi:10.1080/14681994.2020.1749255.

Stefana, A. (2017). Erotic transference. *British Journal of Psychotherapy, 33*(4), 505–513. https://doi-org.proxy.lib.umich.edu/10.1111/bjp.12231.

Taylor, A., & Gosney, M. (2011). Sexuality in older age: Essential considerations for healthcare professionals. *Age ad Ageing, 40,* 538–543. doi:10.1093/ageing/atr049.

Taylor, B., & Davis, S. (2007). The extended PLISSIT model for addressing the sexual wellbeing of individuals with an acquired disability or chronic illness. *Sexual Disability, 25,* 135–139. doi:10.1007/s11195-007-9044-x.

Teyber, E., & Teyber, F. (2017). *Interpersonal process in therapy: An integrative model.* Cengage Learning.

Tuncer, M., & Oskay, Ü. Y. (2022). Sexual counseling with the PLISSIT model: A systematic review. *Journal of Sex & Marital Therapy, 48*(3), 309–318. doi:10.1080/00926 23X.2021.1998270.

Turban, J. (2021). Timing of social transition for transgender and gender diverse youth, K-12 harassment, and adult mental health outcomes. *Journal of Adolescent Health, 69,* 991–998. https://doi.org/10.1016/j.jadohealth.2021.06.001.

Van der Kolk, (2014). *The Body Keeps The Score: Brain, mind, and body in the healing of trauma.* Viking.

Weston, E., & Coleman, E. (2004). Defining sexual health: A descriptive overview. *Archives of Sexual Behavior, 33,* 189–195.

Wilson, P. (2014). *Our whole lives sexuality education for grades 7–9* (2nd Edition). UUA.

Wincze, J., & Weisberg, R. (2015). *Sexual dysfunction: A guide for assessment and treatment* (3rd Edition). Guilford Press.

Workers, N. A. (2008). *NASW code of ethics (guide to the everyday professional conduct of social workers).* NASW.

Index

Note: Page numbers in *italic* indicate a figure and page numbers in **bold** indicate a table on the corresponding page.

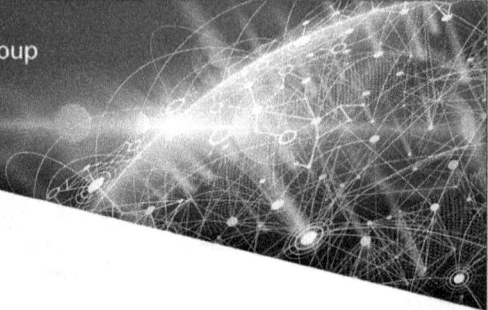

For Product Safety Concerns and Information please contact our EU
representative GPSR@taylorandfrancis.com
Taylor & Francis Verlag GmbH, Kaufingerstraße 24, 80331 München, Germany

www.ingramcontent.com/pod-product-compliance
Lightning Source LLC
Chambersburg PA
CBHW050638280326
41932CB00015B/2701

9 780367 763121